Community Psychiatric Nursing

A research perspective
Volume 3

Edited by

CHARLES BROOKER

Director, Nursing Section
Sheffield Centre for Health and Related Research
UK

and

EDWARD WHITE

Director, Research and Development Unit
Faculty of Health and Social Work
Anglia Polytechnic University
Chelmsford
UK

CHAPMAN & HALL

London · Glasgow · Weinheim · New York · Tokyo · Melbourne · Madras

Published by Chapman & Hall, 2–6 Boundary Row, London SE1 8HN, UK

Chapman & Hall, 2–6 Boundary Row, London SE1 8HN, UK

Blackie Academic & Professional, Wester Cleddens Road, Bishopbriggs, Glasgow G64 2NZ, UK

Chapman & Hall GmbH, Pappelallee 3, 69469 Weinheim, Germany

Chapman & Hall USA, One Penn Plaza, 41st Floor, New York NY 10119, USA

Chapman & Hall Japan, ITP-Japan, Kyowa Building, 3F, 2-2-1 Hirakawacho, Chiyoda-ku, Tokyo 102, Japan

Chapman & Hall Australia, Thomas Nelson Australia, 102 Dodds Street, South Melbourne, Victoria 3205, Australia

Chapman & Hall India, R. Seshadri, 32 Second Main Road, CIT East, Madras 600 035, India

Distributed in the USA and Canada by Singular Publishing Group Inc., 4284 41st Street, San Diego, California 92105

First edition 1995

© 1995 Chapman & Hall

Typeset in 10/12 Times by Mews Photosetting, Beckenham, Kent
Printed in Great Britain by T.J. Press (Padstow) Ltd

ISBN 0 412 59280 0   1 56593 354 0 (USA)

A catalogue record for this book is available from the British Library

Library of Congress Catalog Card Number: 94-69931

∞ Printed on permanent acid-free text paper, manufactured in accordance with ANSI/NISO Z39.48-1992 and ANSI/NISO Z39.48-1984 (Permanence of Paper).

Community Psychiatric Nursing

Contents

Contents

Contributors

Ian Baguley	Clinical Nurse Specialist Tameside Community and Priority Services Trust Ashton-under-Lyne, Greater Manchester
Heather Bartlett	Community Psychiatric Nurse CPN Department Thornbury Day Care Unit London
Joanna Bennett	Lecturer School of Social Work and Health Sciences Middlesex University Enfield, Middlesex
Julia Brooking	formerly Professor of Nursing Studies University of Birmingham Birmingham
Daniel Brown	Clinical Psychology Trainee Institute of Psychiatry London
Anthony Butterworth	Professor of Community Nursing University of Manchester Manchester
Jerome Carson	Lecturer in Clinical Psychology Institute of Psychiatry London

Contributors

Margaret Cooney

Research Associate
Elizabeth Raybold Centre
University of Greenwich
Dartford, Kent

John Done

Principal Lecturer,
Division of Psychology
University of Hertfordshire
Hatfield, Hertfordshire

Leonard Fagin

Consultant Psychiatrist
Claybury Hospital
Woodford Green, Essex

Richard Ford

Head of Service Evaluation
Sainsbury Centre for Mental Health
London

Kevin Gournay

Professor of Mental Health
Middlesex University
Enfield, Middlesex

Phil Harrison-Read

Consultant Psychiatrist
Central Middlesex Hospital
London

Barry Hunt

Head of Division
Pre-registration Adult Nursing
University of Hertfordshire
Hatfield, Hertfordshire

John Leary

Clinical Psychologist
Claybury Hospital
Woodford Green, Essex

Lisa Maclean

Senior Lecturer
Division of Social Work, Counselling,
    Mental Health and Learning Disability
University of Hertfordshire
Hatfield, Hertfordshire

Matt Muijen

Director
Sainsbury Centre for Mental Health
London

Rachel Perkins   Consultant Clinical Psychologist
                        Springfield University Hospital
                        London

Julie Repper   Lecturer
                        Department of Nursing
                        University of Nottingham
                        Nottingham

Monica Savio   PhD student
                        London School of Economics and
                            Political Science
                        London

Geraldine Strathdee   Consultant Community Psychiatrist
                        The Maudsley Hospital
                        London

Edward White   Director, Research and Development
                            Unit
                        Faculty of Health and Social Work
                        Anglia Polytechnic University
                        Chelmsford, Essex

Anne Williams   Senior Lecturer
                        Department of Nursing
                        University of Manchester
                        Manchester

Kate Wilson   Research Officer
                        Health Service Research Unit
                        Department of Public Health and
                            Primary Care
                        University of Oxford
                        Oxford

Foreword

Since the publication of the *Health of the Nation – A Strategy for England*, in 1992, and the adoption of mental illness as one of the five key areas for priority action, mental illness has gained a long overdue share of attention from managers, the media and the general public alike.

The key area handbook for mental illness sets out a framework for the delivery of high quality services which addresses the whole range of mental disorder. Thus, the respective roles of a wide range of agencies, such as primary care, secondary care and the voluntary sector, are outlined within the context of prevention at all levels. Action on key areas includes improving information and understanding about mental illness, the development of local comprehensive services and the dissemination of good clinical practice.

It has become much clearer over recent years that the crucial first step in the commissioning of services is the local assessment of need. This exercise allows high calibre specialist skills to be targeted at those in most need and makes provision for those with less severe problems to be managed by professionals whose skills are more general.

Thus community mental health nurses are a highly skilled specialist workforce, who should be employed to nurse those people suffering from the more severe illness by, for example, carrying out family interventions or assertive case management. There remains an undoubtedly important role to be played in supporting nurses working in primary care settings in their interventions with people with less severe problems such as the milder forms of depression and anxiety which are so common in primary care.

The research reviewed in this book, the third volume of an excellent series, provides both the theoretical and empirical foundation to this basic strategy and is a most timely and authoritative publication which deserves to be read widely by not only mental health nurses but also other mental health professionals, policy makers and purchasers.

Dr R. Jenkins
Principal Medical Officer
Department of Health

Development of a rating scale/checklist to assess the side effects of antipsychotics by community psychiatric nurses

Joanna Bennett, John Done,
Phil Harrison-Read and Barry Hunt

INTRODUCTION

This chapter concerns the second phase of an investigation into community psychiatric nurses' (CPNs) practice with clients on antipsychotic drug therapy. The study focused on the issues of administration of medication and the assessment of clients for side effects.

A number of studies investigating the management of clients with schizophrenia in the community have indicated that better outcomes are achieved with the combination of antipsychotic drug therapy, stress management, skills training and specific psychological interventions (Falloon and Shanahan, 1990; Hogarty *et al.*, 1986; Hogarty and Goldberg, 1974). However, the undesired effects of antipsychotic drugs are often linked with non-compliance with therapy (Hogan, Awad and Eastwood, 1983; Johnson, 1977) and for some clients side effects are as distressing as psychotic symptoms (Finn *et al.*, 1990). Medication side effects are reported to lower clients sociability, the use of leisure time and the quality of personal relationships (Michaels and Mumford, 1989). In addition, it has been shown that fewer medication side effects was one clinical characteristic associated with clients' self-reports of a better quality of life (Sullivan, Wells and Leake, 1992).

It was within this context that the first study, a survey of six CPN teams, was carried out. Data were collected in a number of areas, including the numbers of clients on CPNs' caseloads receiving antipsychotic drugs, the proportion administered and monitored by CPNs, CPNs' knowledge of the side effects of these drugs and their attitude to this aspect of their work. The results of that study showed that CPNs were administering antipsychotic drugs to large numbers of clients in the community and that they reported that they were monitoring these clients frequently for any undesired effects. However, the mean number of side effects CPNs reported they were assessing was three to four per client, done in an unsystematic manner (Bennett, 1991).

The results suggested that, although CPNs reported monitoring clients regularly, they have a limited knowledge of the common side effects of anti-psychotic drugs or that, due to the lack of a systematic method for monitoring them, there is much inconsistency and variability in the CPNs' approach to this area of their work. The results further suggested that CPNs required an improvement in the skills needed to detect and manage the side effects of antipsychotic drugs and that the use of a standardized method would be beneficial.

BACKGROUND

Recent legislation has empowered CPNs to alter the timing and dosage of prescribed drugs used in psychiatry, within a patient-specific protocol. This innovation will therefore require that CPNs have a thorough knowledge of the drugs' action, dosages and side effects (Andrews, 1992) Additionally, they will need to have a full understanding of the assessment and diagnostic process which leads to prescription.

The process of delivering care to clients demands that nurses have the ability to interact well with people and the skills to make physical and psychosocial assessment, implement appropriate interventions and evaluate the outcome of care. The introduction of the nursing process (Marriner, 1979) standard-ized the process of delivering care, with assessment as the initial stage. The areas to be assessed were not specified; therefore strategies and methods may vary between health districts, clinical teams or individual clinicians in the same team.

The first systematic study of the process of assessment in psychiatric nursing was carried out by Gournay, Devilly and Brooker (1993) who used videotapes of assessment interviews to examine the process of community psychiatric nurses' assessment in primary health care. They found that CPNs adopted a client-centred style of approach to assessment, paying little attention to discussing the nature and aims of interventions with clients. The study also showed that CPNs did not use any standard measures in their assessments.

A comprehensive mental health assessment is seen as essential within the framework of the care programme approach, case management and care management of clients with serious mental health problems. To determine the package of care required by each client Ryan, Ford and Clifford (1991), in their evaluation of the outcomes of the RDP (Research and Development for Psychiatry) case management project, have indicated that the assessment and management of medication was an essential component of the clients' package of care.

ASSESSMENT OF THE SIDE EFFECTS OF ANTIPSYCHOTIC DRUGS

The early realization that extrapyramidal side effects (EPs) were generally associated with most antipsychotic drugs led to their assessment being standard practice in the clinical evaluation of these drugs. The main problem with EPs, which are characterized by abnormal involuntary movements or dyskinesias, is that there is no simple method for identifying and measuring their severity. To identify these signs and judge their impact on clients' function requires the clinician to make observations or objective tests, which gives a global impression of the severity of EPs. Standard methods of assessing EPs have developed as a means of evaluating either antipsychotic drugs or different forms of treatment for these disorders.

Standardization of assessment implies that different people using the same measure will obtain similar results. Without such measures, assessment is left to subjective appraisals and the individual's personal judgement. Quantification of symptoms make it possible to report results and changes over time in a more objective and detailed way. In addition, assessing change in a client's condition may involve different clinicians and sharing of information among a multidisciplinary team is easier with standardized measures (Nunnally, 1967). It is now well established that standardization of the psychiatric interview using a clearly defined classification system and rigorous training of raters are essential to making a reliable diagnosis of mental health disorders on which an appropriate intervention can be based.

Two types of assessment have been used to assess medication side effects: subjective assessment based on scales of symptoms and signs or functional disability; and objective tests based on the timing of specific tasks or more complex neurophysiological investigations to measure particular movement disorders (Marsden and Schachter, 1981).

Although a number of standardized methods for assessing extrapyramidal symptoms have been developed for research purposes, the monitoring of EPs and other undesired effects of antipsychotic drugs have not been standardized in routine (or everyday) clinical practice. Reasons include the following.

1. It is often difficult to separate the clinical features of psychopathology, other neurological entities and side effects of antipsychotic drugs.

2. Standardized scales are only available for assessing EPs, which are considered to be the major side effects. These scales and objective tests are often too long or too complicated to administer in clinical practice where there is often limited time and resources.
3. The education/training received by most mental health professionals does not place enough emphasis on the development of skills to detect and manage unwanted effects of medication.
4. Mental health professionals may be reluctant to highlight the negative (iatrogenic) aspects of antipsychotic medication, particularly with the existing problem of maintaining compliance with drug treatment. Instead, the focus is usually on the effectiveness of such drugs in reducing symptoms.

Despite the difficulties and ambiguities, it is clearly necessary to examine ways of integrating the assessment and management of side effects of antipsychotic drugs into the client's package of care, particularly in the case of clients with severe mental disorders requiring long-term maintenance drug therapy in the community. The initial assessment will establish a baseline and allow the rehabilitation team to make informed decisions that take into account all aspects of the client's condition (Lukoff *et al.*, 1992). Assessment of side effects needs to include not only EPs but other common side effects that may affect the client's ability to function and interact socially. In addition, the client's subjective experience of drug therapy should be considered as subjective responses have been associated with non-compliance with medication, poorer clinical outcomes and the presence of akathisia (Van Putten, May and Marder, 1984). Furthermore, other studies have found a positive correlation between clients' self-reports and nursing assessments of side effects (Michaels and Mumford, 1989; Van Putten, 1974).

The evidence outlined above has therefore indicated that there is a need to develop standard methods which can provide valid and reliable screening of clients for common side effects of antipsychotic drugs.

AIMS AND OBJECTIVES

1. To develop an appropriate standard method which CPNs could use in clinical practice to assess clients for side effects of antipsychotic drugs.
2. The schedule should include both the clinician's and the client's assessment of signs and symptoms of abnormal movements and other common side effects.

REVIEW OF EXISTING RATING SCALES

The literature review did not reveal the availability of any reliable standard measures or screening method which covered a wide range of common side effects of antipsychotics. The standard methods available for the assessment of EPs were reviewed. They were thought to be inappropriate for a number of reasons.

Assessment methods based on objective tests, such as peg-board tests, measuring the amplitude of movements and accelerometry, have enormous implications for training and would be too time-consuming and complex for use by CPNs in their clinical practice.

The subjective rating scales of sign and symptoms (e.g. AIMS, TAKES, the Simpson/Rockland tardive dyskinesia rating scale, Smith tardive dyskinesia scale) did not cover the relevant areas to be assessed, as each scale was designed to assess one or at the most two extrapyramidal side effects. Making use of existing scales would entail the selection of two or three scales to cover the range of EPs and in addition the development of an additional schedule that included other common side effects. Such a range of instruments would not be appropriate for use in busy clinical areas or for CPNs with large caseloads.

Finally, in order to maintain the reliability of the existing rating scales they could not be incorporated into the development of a 'side effects scale', with additional items. It was therefore considered appropriate to develop an assessment schedule which included both EPs and other unwanted effects, and which was suitable for clinical practice.

DEVISING THE ITEMS

A rating scale for EPs

Existing rating scales developed to assess EPs and relevant studies of side effects of antipsychotics provided the initial sources of items. The common signs and symptoms of side effects formed the basis for the initial selection of items for the schedule. Once a pool of items had been generated, it was necessary to consider the format of the assessment schedule and the criteria for selection of appropriate items. It was decided that the first part of the assessment should be a rating scale, which would quantify the signs of the movement disorders (dystonia, akathisia, parkinsonism and tardive dyskinesia), to be assessed through a systematic procedure of observing the client. The second part of the assessment should be a checklist of other side effects which are more difficult to observe or quantify, completed by questioning the client. This section should also include items to examine the clients' views on the suitability of their medication.

The criteria for inclusion of items were (1) that clear evidence had shown a particular item to be a sign, symptom or side effect of antipsychotic drugs and (2) that assessment of a particular item could result in some medical or nursing action, i.e. treatment or appropriate management, which would enhance the quality of care received by clients.

A. *Face/mouth/neck*
1. Masked/rigid facial expression (PK)
2. Fixed posture of eyes/neck (D)
3. Increased blinking (TD)
4. Mouth-puckering, pouting or smacking of lips (TD)
5. Abnormal tongue movements (TD)
6. Grimace (TD)

B. *Extremities*
Upper: (arms, hands, fingers)
7. Regular, resting or pill-rolling tremor (PK)
8. Twisting/counting of finger (TD)
Lower: (legs, feet)
9. Shuffling/tapping of feet (AK)

C. *Trunk/posture/gait*
10. Flexed posture (PK)
11. Rocking/shifting or weight/inability to stand still (AK)
12. Twisting/pelvic gyrations (TD)
13. Rigid shuffling gait/reduced arm swing (PK)
14. Slowness of movement (PK)

Part 2. Checklist

Please ask the client the following questions and place a tick in the appropriate box

1. Do you have any of the following: Yes   No   If yes, please
                                                               specify the problem

   a) Dizziness?
   b) Drowsiness?
   c) Sexual problems (ejaculatory, erectile,
      libido, menstrual)?
   d) Constipation?
   e) Urinary problems?
   f) Skin problems (rashes, photosensitivity)?
   g) Excessive weight gain?
   h) Blurred vision?
   i) Feeling restless?
   j) Feeling slow/lethargic?

2. Does the medication agree with you?   Yes/No
   If no, why? (list reasons)

3. Do you think this is the right medication for you?   Yes/No

Figure 1.1 Pre-pilot rating scale/checklist.

Using these parameters, 14 items were selected from the original group to be included in the initial rating scale. The scale was divided into three sections representing body parts: (1) 'Facial/Mouth/Neck', (2) 'Extremities' and (3) 'Trunk'. Each section contained items assessing signs of EPs. One item was selected to assess dystonia (4), five items to assess parkinsonism (PK), two for akathisia (AK) and six items for tardive dyskinesia (TD) (Figure 1.1). The scale items were to be scored on a four point scale of 0–3, according to intensity (0 = absent, 1 = mild, 2 = moderate and 3 = severe).

The signs of agranulocytosis, the main side effect associated with clozapine, were not included in the items selected, as standard procedures are already in place for monitoring clients prescribed this drug.

A client self-report checklist

The second part of the schedule consisted of a list of 10 other common side effects and two items examining appropriateness of medication. With the first 10 items the respondent was asked to answer 'yes' or 'no' and to 'specify the problem' if the response was positive. The final two items requested the client's view on whether the medication agreed with them and whether they felt it was the right medication for them. They were also requested to list the reasons why medication did not 'agree' with them (Figure 1.1).

Inclusion of the final two items was based on studies of clients' subjective response to antipsychotic drugs. One study (Van Putten *et al.*, 1981) used four questions (two similar to those included in this study) to assess the subjective response of clients to antipsychotics. This method of assessment was found to be reliable in dividing clients into those who responded well to medication and those having a 'dysphoric' or negative response. In addition, they found that dysphoric respondents experienced more EPs and that a dysphoric response was a powerful predictor of non-compliance.

MODIFICATION OF THE SCALE/CHECKLIST

Three people with expertise in this area (a psychiatrist, a psychologist and a pharmacologist) were consulted, to ensure unnecessary or ambiguous items were excluded from the scale while ensuring that there were sufficient items to cover the most characteristic signs of the appropriate side effects to be monitored.

The following modifications were made.

The rating scale

Section A

1. The wording of the first item, 'masked/rigid facial expression', was changed to 'unchanging facial expression', a more accurate description of what needed to be rated. Although a rigid facial expression could be indicative of other problems, such as negative symptoms or depression,

a decision was made to include the item, which is important in diagnosing parkinsonism.

2. The second item, 'fixed posture of eyes/neck', was removed, as these signs could be confused with 'abnormal' behaviour (e.g. paranoid behaviour). Additionally, dystonic reaction are on the whole acute reactions to antipsychotic drugs and are seen mainly in the acute setting rather than the community.
3. The item 'increased blinking' was also excluded, as assessing an increased rate would entail establishing the client's normal rate of blinking.
4. Items 4 and 5 assessing abnormal mouth and tongue movements were merged to become 'involuntary movements of mouth, lips or tongue'.
5. The last item in this section, 'grimace', was excluded as it could prove difficult to measure and could be manneristic in origin.

Two items were added to the first section: 'dribbling', a more descriptive term for excessive salivation, a sign of parkinsonism; and 'looks sleepy', which would objectively assess drowsiness.

Section B

Item 8 was excluded as the athetoid movement of the fingers seen with tardive dyskinesia is difficult to separate from individual mannerisms or behaviours due to other psychological processes (e.g. anxiety).

Section C

1. Item 10, 'flexed posture', was removed. Although it may be a sign of parkinsonism, a flexed posture could be indicative of a number of other problems (e.g. depression, a physical disorder).
2. Item 11 was excluded as it was considered ambiguous and the restlessness of akathisia was already covered by another item.
3. The writhing movement, which can affect any part of the body, seen with tardive dyskinesia replaced item 12 'twisting, pelvic gyrations'. In addition to these changes, a category of 'other (please specify)' was added to each section to accommodate clients' individual responses to medication or other atypical variation of unwanted effects (e.g. tremor of the head, noted during this study).

Client's report checklist

There were two changes to this part of the schedule, item 'j' was changed to 'lack get up and go' and an item of 'other' was included, which allowed for individual variation.

Once the format, wording and content of the scale had been agreed, it was necessary to set clear guidelines for rating the intensity of abnormal movements and other items, outline a standard procedure for observing the client and further define some of the items included in the side effects rating scale/checklist. The following assessment procedure and additional definitions of items were adapted from Smith *et al*. (1983).

ASSESSMENT PROCEDURE

Ensure the client has nothing in the mouth (e.g. chewing gum) and, if dentures are worn, that there are no problems with fitting.

Observe client in the following way and complete the rating scale/checklist.

1. Ask the client to sit down; ensure you are an appropriate distance away, so that you can observe hands and feet as well as face. Observe facial and oral movements, also any resting tremor or restlessness of the feet or other parts of the body.
2. Ask the client to open the mouth and then protrude tongue; observe any abnormal tongue movements inside the mouth and when protruding the tongue.
3. Ask the client to stand up while you engage him/her in some conversation; observe posture, trunk including hip movements and any inability to stand still, ask him/her to hold the arms out and observe any hand tremor.
4. Ask the client to walk several paces, turn and walk back twice; observe arm swing and gait.
5. Ask the questions relating to the client's subjective assessment of side effects and the suitability of medication.

ADDITIONAL DEFINITION OF ITEMS

1. **Unchanging facial expression**: rigid-looking face with little spontaneous movement.
3. **Involuntary movements of mouth/lips or tongue**: side-to-side or worm-like rolling and twisting movements of the tongue, puckering, smacking, pouting of lips and mouth.
6. **Pill-rolling**: circular movements of the thumb against index finger.
8. **Tapping of feet/restlessness**: toe tapping, pacing/jogging on the spot.
10. **Pelvic gyrations**: circular or front-to-back movements of the pelvis.
11. **Shuffling gait**: shuffling (dragging) of the feet while walking; knees may be bent.
12. **Reduced arm swing**: arms are fixed or in an unusual position while walking.

Client's subjective assessment

1. c) **Sexual problems**: include erectile/ejaculatory difficulties, menstrual problems and general decreased libido.
    e) **Urinary problems**: include retention or incontinence.
    f) **Skin problems**: include photosensitivity (sunburn) and any rashes.

THE PILOT STUDY

A sample of six CPNs was selected and they were asked to select three clients each ($n = 18$) who were willing to be assessed using the side effects scale/checklist.

Method

The CPNs were each given three schedules, a copy of the assessment procedure, severity ratings and additional definitions of items and an instruction sheet outlining what was required. They were asked to assess each client on one occasion for any side effects using the rating scale/checklist. In addition, they were given a short, four-point questionnaire which asked them to comment firstly on the adequacy of the items in covering the range of side effects of antipsychotics exhibited by clients and to list any items they felt had been omitted; secondly, on the length of time it took to complete assessment; thirdly on the usefulness of such a scale in contributing to the client's overall assessment; and finally, they were asked to make further comments on the scale/checklist.

The procedure for assessment was discussed and any uncertainties regarding severity ratings and definitions of items were clarified. The CPNs were given a period of 2 weeks to select the clients and make the assessments, after which the schedule and questionnaires would be collected. After two visits 15 schedules and five questionnaires were collected.

Results

The responses to the questionnaire showed that the CPNs ($n = 5$) felt that the items on the schedule adequately reflected the types of side effect their clients exhibited and that the schedule made a useful contribution to an overall assessment of clients' needs. The CPNs reported that the mean length of time taken to complete the assessment was 21 minutes. In addition, the following comments were made by the CPNs:

'the scale is a good reminder of side effects to observe for'
'makes for a more detailed assessment'
'definitely an excellent aid'
'useful for monitoring change in side effects'
'consumer perceptions of side effects provided a clearer picture of side effects'.

Although there was no way of checking the reliability of the data collected (Tables 1.1 and 1.2), it was possible to examine the amount of agreement between the clients' report and the CPNs' observations regarding the presence or absence of three items not related to movement disorders. There was 73% level of agreement between clients' reports of 'feeling restless' and 'feeling drowsy' and CPNs' observations of 'restlessness' and 'looking sleepy', and 93% agreement on the report of 'feeling slow' and the CPNs' assessment of 'slowness of movement'.

The CPNs did not suggest any changes to the wording or format of any of the scale/checklist items, possibly because of their lack of experience of standardized methods of assessment. However, the results of the pilot study

Table 1.1 CPNS' assessment

Item	%
Unchanging facial expression	33
Dribbling	27
Involuntary movements of mouth/lips/tongue	44
Looks sleepy	38
Regular resting or pill-rolling tremor	50
Tapping of feet/restlessness	66
Pelvic gyrations or any writhing movements	16
Rigid shuffling gait/reduced arm swing	16
Slowness of movements	61

Table 1.2 Clients' assessment

Item	%
Dizziness	11
Drowsiness	44
Sexual problems	50
Constipation	22
Skin problems	27
Excessive weight gain	38
Feeling restless	55
Lack get up and go	61
Does the medication agree with you? – No	38
Do you think this is the right medication for you? – No	33

showed that: (1) CPNs were able to use a standardized measure to assess their clients for side effects of medication and that they found such a method useful; and (2) the high percentage of agreement between clients' reports and CPNs' assessments indicated that eliciting clients' subjective responses is a valid component of a comprehensive assessment.

The experts (psychiatrist, pharmacologist and psychologist) were again consulted for a final review of the scale/checklist. This resulted in three items being further refined. Item 9, indicating the restlessness of akathisia, was reworded to give clarity and to be more descriptive of the item to be measured. Item 13 was revised to become two items as 'rigid, shuffling gait/reduced arm swing' combined two separate signs of parkinsonism. The final item 'slowness of movements' was changed to 'slowness and reduced spontaneity'.

RESULTS

The final scale/checklist

The final scale contained 14 items, six assessing parkinsonism, two assessing tardive dyskinesia, one assessing akathisia, one assessing oversedation and four assessing other signs not specified within the scale. Although there were only two items assessing tardive dyskinesia, they covered involuntary oral movements and any choreiform or athetoid movements of the trunk or pelvis, the primary symptoms of tardive dyskinesia. In addition, the 'other' categories in the sections assessing extremities allowed for the inclusion of abnormal movements of these areas. These two items were considered adequate to assess tardive dyskinesia, as there is agreement among the experts in this area that subjects with at least one moderate score on an acceptable measure actually have tardive dyskinesia (Whall *et al.*, 1983). Smith *et al.* (1983) have also shown that there is a higher inter-rater reliability with the primary symptoms of tardive dyskinesia than with several unusual symptoms.

The clients' self-report checklist consisted of 13 items: 11 were in the form of a checklist to assess other common side effects and the two global questions remained the same as the draft (Figure 1.2).

Guidelines for rating severity

The initial severity categories of 0–3 (absent, mild, moderate and severe) was expanded to five points of 0–4, with a category of 'uncertain'. This

A. *Face/mouth/neck*
   1. Unchanging facial expression
   2. Dribbling
   3. Involuntary movements of mouth, lips or tongue
   4. Looks sleepy
   5. Other (please specify)

B. *Extremities*
   Upper: (arms, hands, fingers)
   6. Regular, resting or pill-rolling tremor
   7. Other (please specify)
   Lower: (legs, feet)
   8. Tapping of feet/restlessness (jogging on the spot)
   9. Other (please specify)

C. *Trunk/posture/gait*
   10. Pelvic gyrations/or any writhing/rocking movements
   11. Rigid, shuffling gait
   12. Reduced arm swing
   13. Slowness and reduced spontaneity
   14. Other (please specify)

Part 2. Checklist

Please ask the client the following questions and place a tick in the appropriate box
1. Do you have any of the following: Yes   No   If yes, please specify the problem

   a) Dizziness?
   b) Drowsiness?
   c) Sexual problems (ejaculatory, erectile, libido, menstrual)?
   d) Constipation?
   e) Urinary problems?
   f) Skin problems (rashes, photosensitivity)?
   g) Excessive weight gain?
   h) Blurred vision?
   i) Feeling restless?
   j) Lack get up and go?
   k) Other?

2. Does the medication agree with you?   Yes/No
   If no, why? (list reasons)

3. Do you think this is the right medication for you?   Yes/No

Figure 1.2 Final rating/scale checklist.

made allowance for any ambiguity surrounding the underlying cause of 'abnormal' movements or other behaviour. The guidelines also needed to take account of the different criteria needed for rating spontaneous abnormal

Table 1.3 Rating of symptom severity

0	Absent	Signs definitely absent during assessment period
1	Uncertain	Signs may be present but unsure whether they are drug-induced side effects or normal variation, or behaviour resulting from abnormal mental or other cause
2	Mild	Signs just detectable and, in the case of spontaneous abnormal movements, present only occasionally
3	Moderate	Signs moderate or, in the case of spontaneous abnormal movements, pronounced but present only occasionally or mild but present most or all of the time
4	Severe	Signs pronounced and, in the case of spontaneous abnormal movements, present most or all of the time

movements versus other items; thus the guidance for rating severity set out in Table 1.3 was developed.

Once the scale/checklist, the guidelines for rating severity, the additional definition of items and the assessment procedure were finalized, it was necessary to test the reliability of the scale, i.e. whether independent raters could agree on a score when rating a client at the same time.

Inter-rater reliability

It was decided that the use of video recordings of subjects would be more acceptable in ethical terms than using live subjects. One problem with the videotaping technique is that movements are reduced to two dimensions, which may make them more difficult to identify. Despite this problem the audio-visual technique is widely used for training purposes and evaluating drug effects (Gardos and Cole, 1980).

A consultant psychiatrist with expertise in psychopharmacology and previous experience of using audio-visual techniques in drug evaluation studies collaborated with this phase of the study.

Method

Ten clients were videotaped in three sessions of 2–3 hours. The clients were selected from an acute psychiatric unit by the consultant psychiatrist after giving a brief explanation of the study and receiving a verbal consent. The clients were then escorted to a separate room and, prior to videotaping, a more detailed explanation was given regarding the psychiatrist's assessment, the study, the possible uses of the recording and the client's right to have the tape destroyed at any time. The clients were assured that their identity and any information obtained would be confidential. They were then asked to sign a consent form.

Each client was then recorded as he/she was assessed by the psychiatrist, following the procedure outlined above. Firstly the client was asked to sit in an upright chair with their feet squarely on the floor and hands relaxed on the lap while the psychiatrist, also sitting, discussed any problems the clients had that they perceived to be side effects of their medication. During this period the video recording focused for about 1–2 minutes on the client's feet, to record any restless movements, the hands, to record any resting tremor, and the mouth for oral movements. The client was then asked by the psychiatrist to open the mouth and protrude the tongue. The mouth was recorded to capture any abnormal movements.

The client was then asked to stand and, while the psychiatrist engaged him/her in conversation, the client's feet were recorded for any restless movements and the whole body to enable observation of posture and any trunk or hip movements.

Finally the client was asked to walk normally several times across the room; this recording enabled observation of gait and arm swing.

In collaboration with the psychiatrist, six clients were selected and edited as appropriate examples of clients exhibiting most of the items on the rating scale at varying degrees of severity. The length of the final video was 25 minutes. There were no examples of dribbling and pelvic gyrations, as none of the clients recorded exhibited these signs.

Four research colleagues were requested to observe the recordings of the six clients and give ratings using the scale. The raters were from different professional backgrounds (two psychologists, a pharmacologist and a psychiatric nurse) but all were familiar with movement disorders through previous research studies or clinical practice. Time was allocated for the raters to read the guidelines for rating severity and clarify any issues that might arise.

Statistical analysis

The Pearson r was used to calculate the correlation coefficients between the four raters. To determine the overall association the mean of these coefficients was computed, as the number of raters was small (Siegel, 1956). A critical values table for the Pearson r was used (Fisher and Yates, 1974), to test the null hypothesis that $p = 0$, ensuring that the correlation coefficient obtained was not due merely to chance.

The following items were excluded from the analysis of inter-rater reliability: items 2 and 10, 'dribbling' and 'pelvic gyrations/or any writhing rocking movement', as the test videotape did not include examples of these items and none of the four raters had given a score for them. In addition, items 5, 7, 9 and 14, the categories of 'other', were excluded, as these were used infrequently and the signs identified and scored were not consistent across raters.

Results

The inter-rater reliability for the scale was $r = 0.82$, significant at $p < 0.05$, calculated using the total score for each item. Reliabilities for the individual scale items were also calculated. Table 1.4 shows the mean correlation coefficients for the eight items.

Table 1.4 Correlation coefficients between raters ($n = 6$)

	Mean	*Range*
1. Unchanging facial expression	0.34	−0.333–0.962
3. Involuntary movements of mouth, lips or tongue	0.21	−0.522–0.905
4. Looks sleepy	0.34	−0.333–1.000
6. Regular, resting or pill-rolling tremor	−0.11	−0.333–0.577
8. Tapping of feet/restlessness (jogging on the spot)	0.70*	0.471–0.866
11. Rigid, shuffling gait	0.83*	0.725–1.000
12. Reduced arm swing	0.83*	0.725–1.000
13. Slowness and reduced spontaneity	0.90*	0.818–0.986

*Significant at $p = 0.05$ or below

The reliabilities for the three parkinsonian items and for restlessnes (akathisia) were also high and significant at $p < 0.05$. The mean correlations between the raters of involuntary mouth and tongue movements, facial expression, drowsiness and tremor were considerably lower. However, as the clients that were rated had only mild levels of these side effects, the range of scores from perfect to negative correlations between raters showed that even some experienced raters found it difficult to detect the early signs of some side effects. Of particular importance is involuntary mouth movements, an early sign of tardive dyskinesia. A parkinsonian subscale was derived from five items: 'unchanging facial expression', 'regular, resting or pill-rolling tremor', 'rigid shuffling gait', 'reduced arm swing' and 'slowness and reduced spontaneity'. The mean correlation between the four raters for the subscale was calculated using total score for each of the five items. The parkinsonian subscale scores showed a statistically significant correlation ($r = 0.81$, $p < 0.05$, range 0.618–0.995).

DISCUSSION

This initial study has shown that the reliability of the rating scale was quite high with experienced untrained raters. The correlations were consistently high for the total scale (0.82), for the parkinsonian subscale (0.81), for the four individual parkinsonian items and for restlessness (akathisia). The lower reliabilities for some individual items, i.e. unchanging facial expression, tremor, looking sleepy (drowsiness) and involuntary mouth and tongue movements, may be due to the difficulty in distinguishing these signs and symptoms from normal or psychopathological behaviours, particularly if they are mild in severity. As the test video contained only examples of mild symptoms, it may have been difficult for raters to detect them on a video recording. The lower reliabilities obtained for some individual items are consistent with the results obtained in similar studies (e.g. Smith *et al.*, 1983).

It was difficult to identify clients with moderate or severe examples of these symptoms, possibly because of the use of lower doses of antipsychotics and treatment with anticholinergic and other drugs. Mild signs of tremor, unchanging facial expression and drowsiness may not affect the client's functioning or be of importance in managing medication (e.g. compliance). However, it is important that CPNs are able to detect involuntary mouth movements, an early sign of tardive dyskinesia.

As the correlation coefficient for involuntary mouth and tongue movements as an individual item was low (0.21), future raters will require specific training on the rating of this item. In addition, a training programme will need to include examples of writhing and rocking movements, to enable CPNs to rate this item should a client exhibit such symptoms.

Correlations were not calculated for the four individual items of 'other', but are important in clinical practice to identify individual variation of symptoms.

This study has shown that CPNs, even though untrained in the use of the outlined schedule, reported that it was useful in making a comprehensive assessment of their clients for side effects and monitoring change over time. Additionally, there was a high level of agreement between CPNs' assessment and clients' reports of some items.

The study has also highlighted the important stages in development of a measurement scale. The initial reliability study has demonstrated that it is possible to devise a reliable rating scale consisting of the key clinical signs and symptoms of the common side effcts of antipsychotics. However, although high reliability has been obtained for the scale and some individual items, there is an indication that training is necessary to enable raters to detect milder symptoms.

FURTHER DEVELOPMENTS

Although not reported here, it may be of interest to note how this study has continued. A training programme was developed which included videotaped examples of all the signs and symptoms of movement disorders included in the scale. A group of CPNs were trained to use the scale/checklist and were subsequently required to use it to assess a selected number of their clients for a 3-month period. These CPNs were compared with a control group of CPNs on a number of variables, to assess the effects of training and the benefits of using the scale in clinical practice.

REFERENCES

Andrews, S. (1992) Prescription for success. *Health Direct*, **March**, 12.

Bennett, J. (1991) Drugs and the CPN. *Nursing Times*, **44**, 38–40.

Falloon, R.H. and Shanahan, W. (1990) Community management of schizophrenia. *British Journal of Hospital Medicine*, **43**, 62–5.

Finn, S.E., Bailey, J.M., Schultz, R.T. and Faber, R. (1990) Subjective utility ratings of neuroleptics in treating schizophrenia. *Psychological Medicine*, **20**, 843–8.

Fisher, R.A. and Yates, F. (1974) *Statistical Tables for Biological, Agricultural and Medical Research*. Longman, London.

Gardos, G. and Cole, J.O. (1980) Problems in the assessment of tardive dyskinesia, in *Tardive Dyskinesia: Research and Treatment*, (ed. W.E. Fann *et al.*), Spectrum, New York.

Gournay, K.J.M., Devilly, G. and Brooker, C. (1993) The CPN in primary care: a pilot study of the process of assessment, in *Community Psychiatric Nursing – A Research Perspective*, vol. 2, (eds C. Brooker and E. White), Chapman & Hall, London.

Hogan, T.P., Awad, A.G. and Eastwood, R. (1983) A self-report scale predictive of drug compliance in schizophrenics: reliability and discriminative validity. *Psychological Medicine*, **13**, 177–83.

Hogarty, G.E. and Goldberg, S.C. (1974) Drug and sociotherapy in the aftercare of schizophrenic patients. *Archives of General Psychiatry*, **28**, 54–64.

Hogarty, G.W., Anderson, C.M., Reiss, D.J. *et al.* (1986) Family psychoeducation, social skills training and maintenance chemotherapy in the aftercare treatment of schizophrenia. *Archives of General Psychiatry*, **43**, 633–42.

Johnson, D.A.W. (1977) Practical considerations in the use of depot neuroleptics for the treatment of schizophrenia. *British Journal of Hospital Medicine*, **June**, 546–58.

Lukoff, D., Ventura, J., Nuechterlein, K. and Liberman, R.P. (1992) Integrating symptom assessment into psychiatric rehabilitation, in *Handbook of Psychiatric Rehabilitation* (ed. R.P. Liberman), Maxwell Macmillan, Oxford.

Marriner, A. (1979) *The Nursing Process*. C.V. Mosby, St Louis.

Marsden, C.D. and Schachter, M. (1981) Assessment of extrapyramidal disorders. *British Journal of Clinical Pharmacology*, **11**, 129–51.

Michaels, R.A. and Mumford, K. (1989) Identifying akinesia and akathisia: the relationship between patient's self-report and nurse's assessment. *Archives of Psychiatric Nursing*, **3**, 97–101.

Nunnally, J.C. (1967) *Psychometric Theory*, McGraw-Hill, New York.

Ryan, P., Ford, R. and Clifford, P. (1991) *Case Management and Community Care*, Research and Development for Psychiatry, London.

Siegel, S. (1956) *Nonparametric Statistics for the Behavioural Sciences*. McGraw-Hill, New York.

Smith, R.C., Allen, R.A., Gordon, J. and Wolff, J. (1983) A rating scale for tardive dyskinesia and parkinsonian symptoms. *Psychopharmacology Bulletin*, **19**, 267–75.

Sullivan, G., Wells, K.B. and Leake, B. (1992) Clinical factors associated with better quality of life in a seriously mentally ill population. *Hospital and Community Psychiatry*, **43**, 794–9.

Van Putten, T. (1974) Why do schizophrenic patients refuse to take their drugs? *Archives of General Psychiatry*, **31**, 67–72.

Van Putten, T., May, P.R.A. and Marder, S.R. (1984) Responses to antipsychotic medication: the doctor's and the consumer's view. *American Journal of Psychiatry*, **141**, 116–19.

Van Putten, T., May, P.R.A., Marder, S.R. and Wittmann, L.A. (1981) Subjective response to antipsychotic drugs. *Archives of General Psychiatry*, **38**, 187–90.

Whall, A.L., Engle, V., Edwards, A. *et al.* (1983) Development of a screening program for tardive dyskinesia: feasibility issues. *Nursing Research*, **32**, 151–6.

CHAPTER TWO

The community psychiatric nurse in primary care: an economic analysis

Kevin Gournay and Julia Brooking

INTRODUCTION

While health economics has a literature which goes back many years, our ability to make service allocation choices on both clinical and economic grounds remains extremely limited.

A major review of economic evaluations of mental health care was conducted by O'Donnell, Maynard and Wright (1988). The authors argued that because mental health care resources are so scarce, making choices between alternative claims on these resources is unavoidable. Thus the most efficient use of these resources must be identified and chosen by a process of collecting information on the costs and benefits of alternative modes of care. The authors pointed out that there was very little evidence of the efficacy of alternative programmes and that despite the very long-standing policy decision to shift care into the community, there was at that time very little evidence of the resource consequences of such change. More recently, however, there have been some studies conducted into service provision and the TAPS project in North East Thames Regional Health Authority (Knapp *et al.*, 1990; Leff, 1993) and the comparison of intensive community care versus traditional inpatient care within the context of the Daily Living Programme (Muijen, Marks and Connolly, 1992) are good exemplars. However, the point made by O'Donnell and his colleagues that most therapies and policies are unevaluated remains valid. Furthermore, these therapies and policies are maintained not because of demonstrable efficiency but because of received wisdom and customary practice. In conclusion, the authors state unequivocally that such inefficient behaviour is both unscientific and unethical.

Before reviewing the specific literature relating to mental health nursing, one development in the application of health economics in mental health is worth noting, if only to emphasize the importance and changing nature of this area. Wilkinson *et al.* (1990) were the first to examine the possibility of transferring a widely used methodology of health economics in medicine to psychiatry. In particular, they conducted a pilot study of the use of the Quality Adjusted Life Year (QALY) in a psychiatric setting. To recap, the QALY uses ratings of disability and distress. One way of describing health status is the Rosser scale (Rosser and Kind, 1978; Rosser and Watts, 1972) (Table 2.1).

Table 2.1 Rosser's classification of illness states

Disability	Distress
1. No disability	a. No distress
2. Slight social disability	b. Mild
3. Severe social disability and/or slight impairment of performance at work Able to do all housework except very heavy tasks	c. Moderate d. Severe
4. Choice of work or performance at work very severely limited Housewives and old people able to do light housework only but able to go out shopping	
5. Unable to take any paid employment Unable to continue any education Old people confined to home except for escorted outings and short walks and unable to do shopping Housewives able only to perform a few simple tasks	
6. Confined to chair or able to move around in the house only with support from an assistant	
7. Confined to bed	
8. Unconscious	

This study was carried out in Buckingham on a sample of 14 men and 24 women with predominant diagnoses of schizophrenia (15), affective disorder (13) and neurosis (10). The authors used three measures, a clinical global impression scale, a quality of life measure and a frequency measure of number of contacts with professionals by subjects. The study looked at the cost of intervention with these subjects, where the main foci of intervention were the prevention of further episodes of mental ill health and an improvement in social function. Simple calculation showed that the costs per QALY were lowest with people with schizophrenia and highest with those with neurotic disorder. However, the authors pointed out that although it should, in principle, be easy to translate QALY comparisons between competing psychiatric programmes, there were two major problems. First they pointed out that the QALY approach and the associated values in the Rosser matrix still emphasized the extension of life and that in mental health programmes this is rarely an aim. However, since that time the values in the Rosser matrix have been updated, based on a larger and more representative sample, and much greater weight has been attached to improvement in health state and particularly improvement in mental health (Gudex *et al.*, 1993). This more recent modification therefore puts psychiatry into a more equitable position as far as comparison with medical and surgical treatments. Secondly, the authors point to other work which shows that there are problems in measuring the sort of specific disability and distress found in mental disorders. This therefore leads to the position that the health status of patients with mental health problems is probably not accurately measured. The authors concluded by stating that, while psychiatry has much to gain from the development of objective and standard measures for comparing programmes, QALYs have yet to prove that they can fill that role. However, given the changes in calculations referred to above, this conclusion may need to be somewhat reconsidered.

Additionally, a recent monograph by Culyer and Wagstaff (1992) argues convincingly that QALYs have yet to be bettered by the more recent measure the Healthy Year Equivalent (Gafni, 1989; Mehrez and Gafni, 1989). It should also be pointed out that the Wilkinson *et al.* study, albeit a useful preliminary piece of work, had three flaws. First the numbers of patients were relatively small, secondly, there was no control group and third, there was no baseline period which might have demonstrated whether patients would remain in their initial state without intervention.

CPNs AND COST EFFECTIVENESS

There have been numerous suggestions over the years that CPN attachments in PHC may be very cost effective. Indeed Illing *et al.* (1990), in their evaluation of CPNs in general practice, placed considerable emphasis on the possibility that CPNs may save money. Indeed, the authors asserted that this saving was effected by diverting patients away from more expensive treatments, i.e. referral to outpatients and admission to hospital. They also described the likelihood that CPN intervention would reduce GP prescribing. However, none of these assertions were based on any controlled enquiry.

Prior to the current study there were only two British controlled economic analyses of mental health nursing. The first was that of the Springfield

Research Team (Paykel and Griffith, 1983; Mangen *et al.*, 1983) who showed that CPNs were more expensive in direct costs in the first 6 months of follow-up because of increased contacts. However, thereafter and in the 18 months of the study as a whole, CPN care was cheaper. With regard to the overall costs of psychiatric services there were no significant differences between the CPN group and the group followed up by psychiatrists. Furthermore there was no overall difference between the two groups in the cost of psychotropic medication. The authors suggested that the relative cheapness of the CPN follow-up condition may well continue and become more marked in the period after the 18 months of the study.

In the only controlled economic analysis of mental health nursing in PHC, Ginsberg, Marks and Waters (1984) looked at the economic outcome of patients treated with behaviour therapy by nurse therapists. (This economic analysis was carried out within the setting of the controlled study of Marks, 1985.) The study compared these patients with a group of patients receiving routine GP care. The work built heavily on a previous uncontrolled study of 42 out-patients with adult neurotic problems treated by nurse therapists (Ginsberg and Marks, 1977). This previous work showed a decreased resource use after nurse therapy intervention and Marks argued convincingly that the benefits to the community would continue over the years. In the Ginsberg, Marks and Waters (1984) study there were only modest savings in the nurse therapy treatment condition and the authors drew attention to the relatively incomplete data returned by the patient sample. Ginsberg and his colleagues therefore claimed that their conclusions must be tempered with caution. However, they also argued that if one assumed that nurse therapists treated more than the 39 patients per year described in the study and if treatment gains continued beyond the 2-year follow-up period, then there would be considerable benefits to the patient and to society. The first assumption is based on considerable available data (e.g. Brooker and Brown, 1986; Gournay and Newell, 1993) which show that nurse therapists tend to treat more than this figure of 39 patients a year. Regarding the second assumption, the authors cited considerable evidence to show that patients with phobias and obsessive compulsive disorder maintained their gains at follow-up periods of up to 7 years. Marks (1985), in the conclusion of his monograph, suggested that a nurse therapist could be fully occupied working with 12 general practitioners serving a population of 30 000 people. He estimated that this would enable the nurse therapist to meet most of the specific need for behaviour therapy of PHC patients in their catchment population.

METHOD

This economic evaluation was carried out within the context of a controlled study carried out between 1988 and 1991. The full results of the outcome study are reported elsewhere (Gournay and Brooking, 1992, 1994).

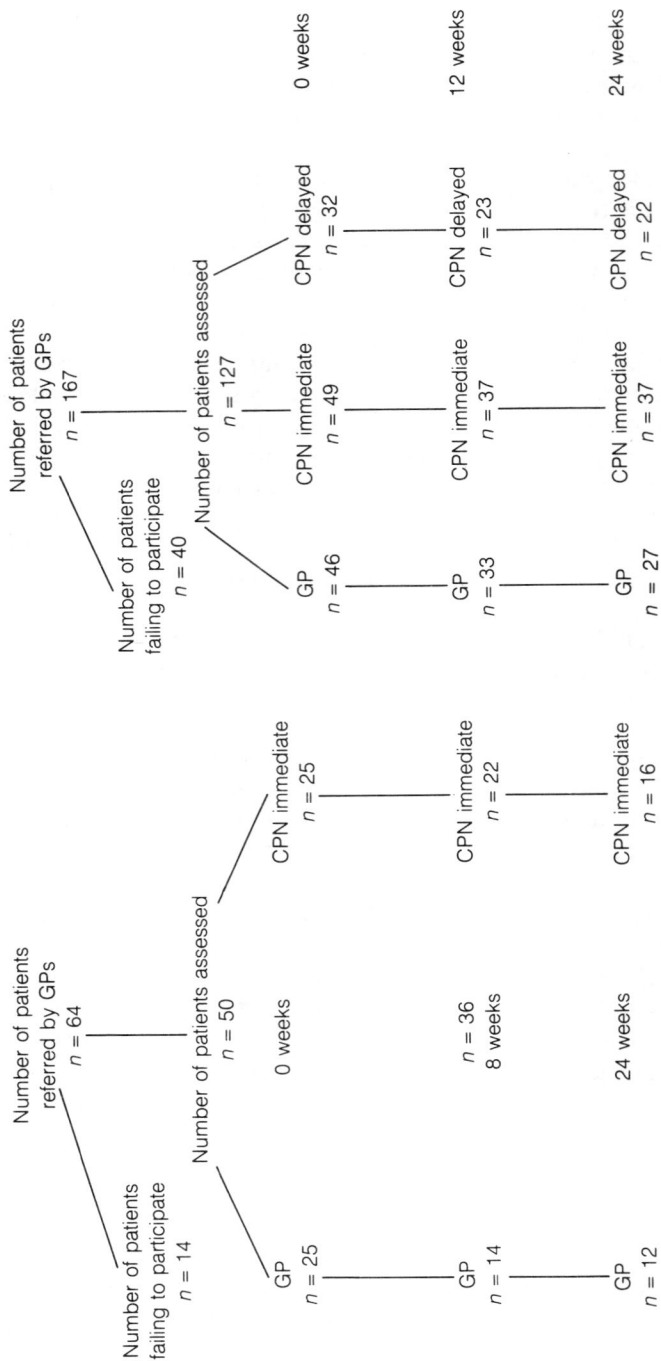

Figure 2.1 Patient flow (numbers indicate patients who completed research assessment).

In summary, the study looked at 11 CPNs working in six primary care settings in two North London health authorities (Barnet and Parkside). Patients suffering a range of non-psychotic problems were randomly allocated in two phases to one of three conditions: (1) immediate CPN intervention (2) CPN intervention, delayed for 12 weeks, or (3) continuing GP care. See Figure 2.1 for detail of patient flow. Outcome was assessed by a variety of measures of change (see below). We also examined aspects of the structure and process of CPN work in this area, but this is reported elsewhere, (Gournay, Devilly and Brooker, 1993).

As the graphs show (Figure 2.2), the patients showed significant improvement (on the measures) over time. But there were no differences between the group receiving CPN intervention and that receiving routine GP care. In addition we found that 50% of patients dropped out of CPN intervention. Furthermore there was no relationship between clinical improvement and the amount of contact with the CPN. As only eight patients in the delayed condition remained in contact with the CPN (although we did assess dropouts as well) we have not shown this group's results in Figure 2.2.

DESIGN AND METHOD OF ECONOMIC STUDY

Much of our methodology is based on that used in the studies of Ginsberg, Marks and Waters (1984) and Mangen *et al*. (1983).

Categories of cost

Categories of cost about which data were collected were as follows:

1. patients' absences from work;
2. drugs and dispensing;
3. use of non-psychiatric hospital treatment resources;
4. use of all GP resources;
5. use of all CPN resources;
6. use of other psychiatric treatment resources;
7. use of local authority social services;
8. social security rent and rebate (transfer payments);
9. patients' and relatives' travel and work loss for treatment;
10. patients' personal expenses;
11. relatives' work losses and other costs incurred because of the patient's problem.

Data collection

We collected data as follows:

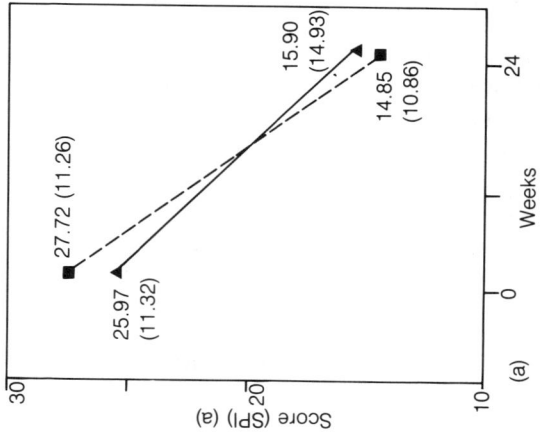

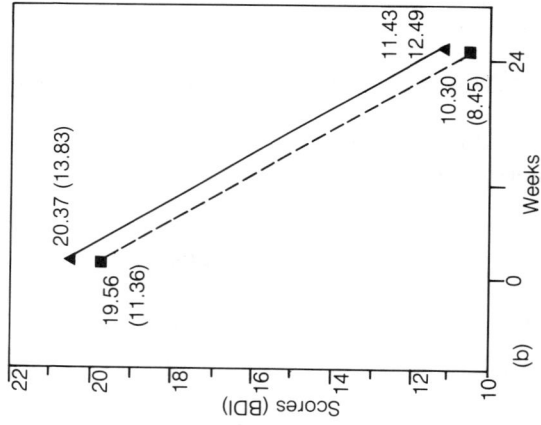

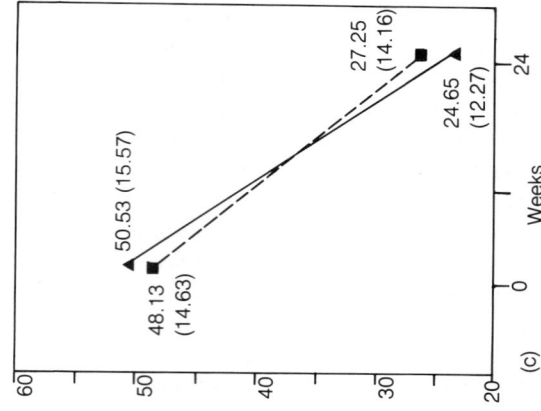

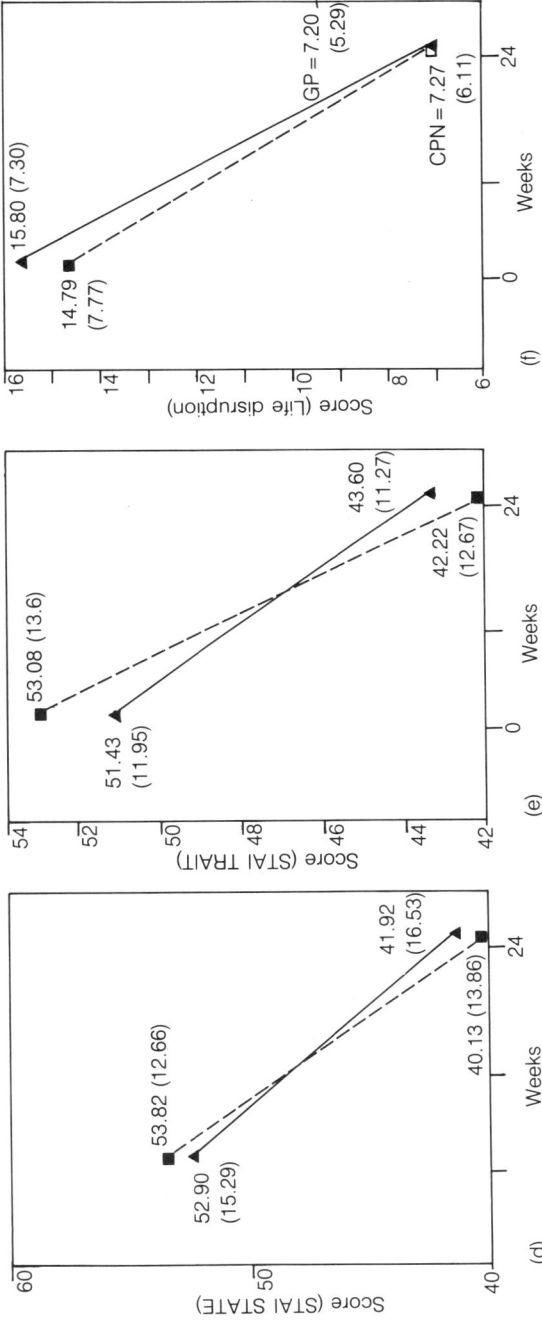

Figure 2.2 Scores on measures for patients allocated to CPN intervention or continuing GP care: **(a)** Standardized Psychiatric Interview; **(b)** Beck Depression Inventory; **(c)** General Health Questionnaire; **(d)** Spielberger State Anxiety; **(e)** Spielberger Trait Anxiety; **(f)** Life disruption/scores. ▲ = CPN; ■ = GP. For all measures, differences between groups are not significant; differences between rating points $p < 0.001$.

1. patients' GP and CPN records yielded data about GP visits, CPN sessions and drug usage;
2. all patients who consented were interviewed using an economic question-naire (EQ).

Rating points

The EQ was used at entry into the study (for cost data prior to intervention) and at 24 weeks follow-up (for cost data for the intervention period).

Economic questionnaire

This was the main instrument of our study and was based on that used by Ginsberg, Marks and Waters (1984). Amendments to the EQ as used by Ginsberg, Marks and Waters were as follows.

1. All time periods refer to 6 months rather than 12 months as our research design allowed for only a 6-month follow-up period.
2. Resource usage by patients was noted for whatever reason. The EQ of Ginsberg *et al.* emphasized 'due to your problem' in a number of cases. We felt that this specificity created difficulties as reasons for attending one's GP are often unclear or multiple in nature.
3. Information concerning Social Security benefits also included rent rebate payments.
4. A clear distinction was made between psychiatric inpatient care and non-psychiatric inpatient care. If patients had inpatient treatment, the location and reasons for it were also ascertained.
5. Questions referring to the behaviour of patients' children due to patients' problems were omitted as these data were not directly relevant to our research questions.

Basic costing procedure

For each patient the costing of the categories outlined previously was as follows.

1. *Patients' absences from work*: The costing of absences from work included time off sick or periods of unemployment due to any problems (psychiatric or physical). The production loss was valued at the patients' salary for that period. In 1988 average productivity was estimated to be £65 per day (see below and Table 2.2). These data were obtained via our Economic Adviser at the Department of Health.

Table 2.2 Examples of unit costs used in the economic analysis (based on the most up-to-date figures available at commencement of data collection in 1988)

	Cost(£)
Community Psychiatric Nurse	8.96/hour
General Practitioner	52.01/hour
Practice Nurse	6.23/hour
General Hospital Outpatient	30.21/attendance
General Hospital Daypatient	82.57/day
General Hospital Inpatient	110.47/day
Physiotherapy	8.43/hour
Dietitian	8.43/hour
Psychiatric Outpatient	42.03/attendance
Social Worker	11.36/hour
Social Worker (home visit)	11.97/hour
Clinical Psychologist	9.31/hour
Average productivity	65.00/day

2. *Drugs and dispensing*: Records of drug prescriptions were taken (where possible) from GP records and costed according to prices stated in the Monthly Index of Medical Specialities for January 1988.
3. *Use of non-psychiatric treatment resources*: Patients were asked to report on the number of days spent as an inpatient in general hospitals and number of outpatient and day patient attendances. These were costed according to the unit costs for each service.
4. *Use of GP resources*: This included the number of visits to the GP and the length of session, together with any domiciliary visits from a GP. These were costed according to the figures shown in Table 2.2.
5. *Use of CPN resources*: Number of sessions and the length of session with the CPNs were ascertained, together with any travelling expenses incurred.
6. *Use of other psychiatric treatment resources*: Length and number of sessions with any other psychiatric services; inpatient and day patient care at psychiatric hospitals/units were also recorded and costed.
7. *Local authority and social service resources*: Services provided by local authority social services (e.g. meals on wheels, hostels, child care) were recorded.
8. *Social Security, rent and rebate payments*: All these transfer payments were recorded.
9. *Patients' and relatives' travel and work loss due to treatment*.
10. *Patients' personal expenses*: Any expenses incurred by patients for private health care treatment, privately employed childminders or home help support were documented.

Table 2.3 Cost data for experimental groups at assessment and 24-week follow-up

Category	CPN (n = 49)		GP (n = 46)	
	0 weeks	24 weeks	0 weeks	24 weeks
Absences from work (days) (mean for all patients)	a.* 10.97 b.** 9.57	6.87 5.35	10.64 8.03	10.87 10.21
Drugs and dispensing (no. of patients receiving prescriptions for psychotropics)	4	9	3	11
Non-psychiatric treatment (total inpatient days for all patients)	13	14	14	14
GP resources (mean cost in £ for all patients)	56.82	43.42	68.91	39.53
CPN resources (mean cost in £ for all patients)	–	48.17	–	–
Other psychiatric treatment resources (£)	336.24	233.09 (for 4 patients)	378.27	126.09 (for 2 patients)
Local authority and social service resources (£)	–	249.92 (social worker for 2 patients)	–	159.04 (social worker for 2 patients)
Social Security payments (mean total £ over 6-month period)	1644 mean for 11 patients	1647	1356 mean for 12 patients	1307
Patients' and relatives' work loss and travel cost (all patients)				
mean cost (£)	–	0.66	–	0.57
distance in miles (car drivers)	–	2.2	–	1.7
Patients' other expenses (private treatment etc.) (£)	63.00 (mean for 3 patients)	219.20 (mean for 7 patients)	158.00 (mean for 3 patients)	182.00 (mean for 6 patients)

*all absences **for presenting problem

11. *Relatives' work losses due to problem of patients*: Although patients' relatives did not participate, patients were asked whether their relatives incurred expenditure as a result of caring for the patient.

Costings used in the study

Table 2.2 shows the unit costs used in the economic analysis. As the data collection of the study was spread over 2½ years we have used, for simplicity, the costs at the time of commencement of the study in 1988.

RESULTS

We excluded data from patients in the CPN delayed group because of the addition of the CPN intervention between rating points. A summary of cost data is shown in Table 2.3.

Absences from work

Table 2.3 shows changes in absences of work broken down by whether the absence was because of the presenting problem or for other reasons.

The change in absence rates (for both categories) showed a statistically significant reduction over time for the CPN condition ($p < 0.01$), with patients in this group having on average slightly more than 4 days less off work over the 6 months of the study than over the previous 6 months.

Using the unit costs referred to in Table 2.2 the net saving per patient (over the time period of the study) in the CPN condition was £267 compared with a net increase for the GP condition of £15 (Table 2.4).

Drugs

We were able to access computerized drug records for 114 patients. One practice in our sample was unable to provide us with any information.

A total of 27 patients received prescriptions for psychotropic medication (13 in the CPN condition and 14 in the GP condition). Of the 13 patients in the CPN condition, four dropped out of CPN intervention.

Of the 14 patients in the GP condition, three received prescriptions for hypnotics (all benzodiazepines) alone; 11 patients received prescriptions for antidepressant medication. Eight of the 11 also received prescriptions for benzodiazepine hypnotics, benzodiazepine tranquillizers or (two patients)

Table 2.4 Net cost per patient (£) of CPN and GP treatment group (negative net costs represent net benefit; all costs rounded to nearest £)

	CPN			GP		
	Before	After	Net cost	Before	After	Net cost
Work absences	713	447	−267	692	707	15
Drugs	–	–	–	–	–	–
Non-psychiatric treatment	–	4	4	–	–	0
GP resources	57	43	−13	69	40	−29
Other psychiatric treatment resources	7	5	−2	8	3	−5
Local authority and social services resources	–	5	5	–	3	3
Social Security	–	–	–	–	–	−13
Other	1	4	3	3	4	1
Total			−270			−29
CPN resources		48	48			
Total net cost			−221			−29
Net cost of CPN option			−193			

a phenothiazine. Of these 14 patients, three only received prescriptions for psychotropic drugs in the 6 months before the initial referral to the study and assessment.

Of the 13 patients in the CPN condition, three received prescriptions for benzodiazepine hypnotics alone and one patient received a prescription for a non-benzodiazepine hypnotic. Nine patients received prescriptions for antidepressant medication. Six of these nine also received prescriptions for benzodiazepine hypnotics and (one patient) a phenothiazine. Of these 13 patients, four only received prescriptions in the 6 months before the initial referral to the study and assessment.

Therefore, in terms of numbers of patients receiving psychotropic drugs there were no differences between the two conditions either before or during the study.

Careful scrutiny of individual records shows that the issue of drug treatment is complex and some examples may help to demonstrate this.

Two patients in the GP condition received prescriptions for expensive drugs such as lofepramine hydrochloride (cost in MIMS £44.50 for 250 tablets) and, while numbers of prescriptions were similar for the experimental groups, prescriptions for more expensive drugs obviously distort cost calculations.

Antidepressant medication was rarely prescribed for much longer than 2 months and sometimes in very low doses (e.g. imipramine 10 mg o.n.). Most patients received doses (e.g. amitriptyline 50 mg o.n.) that would be considered as subtherapeutic by most experts (Deakin, 1986).

To ensure that prescribing had no major influence on the outcome results, outcome data for subjects receiving prescriptions were subjected to analysis. In the event outcome was similar for these two small groups and therefore this phenomenon had no bearing on the major results of our study.

Non-psychiatric treatment

As Table 2.3 shows, inpatient days (in a mixture of private and NHS hospitals) for non-psychiatric complaints was virtually identical for both groups over time.

We are unable to report data on outpatient or day patient attendances for non-psychiatric complaints.

GP resources

GP consultant times were extracted from the economic questionnaire data; therefore the costings can only be approximate. There were no differences in GP consultation times for patients in the CPN condition and patients in the GP condition.

As Table 2.5 shows, reduction in GP consultations for the patients in the GP condition was statistically significant.

Table 2.5 Comparison of consultation rates for all patients during the study period and in the 6 months before the study

	No. GP consultations in 6 months before study (SD)	*No. GP consultations in 6 months of study (SD)*
GP condition ($n = 39$)	5.30*(4.01)	3.04*(2.84)
CPN immediate condition (all) ($n = 53$)	4.37(3.46)	3.34(2.93)
CPN immediate condition (continuers/completers) ($n = 33$)	3.00**(1.55)	3.25(1.82)
CPN immediate condition (dropouts) ($n = 20$)	5.35**(3.75)	3.50(2.82)

*significant over time $p < 0.05$; **significant between $p < 0.05$. Difference between GP condition and CPN condition n.s.

CPN resources

Costings were based on a mean session length of 58 minutes. No other CPN contact was reported for the GP group or for the CPN group in the 6 months before the initial assessment.

Other psychiatric treatment resources

As Table 2.3 shows, in the 6 months prior to the study, eight patients in the CPN condition and nine patients in the GP condition attended a psychiatric outpatients clinic.

For the 6 months of the study, two patients in the GP condition attended psychiatric outpatients for a total of three sessions. Three patients in the CPN condition attended psychiatric outpatients, each for an assessment only. One patient in the CPN condition received a domiciliary visit from the crisis intervention service (this team consisted of a psychiatric registrar and a social worker). Costs were based on the assumption of 2 hours of investment by this team.

Local authority and social services resources

None of the patients in the study reported use of local authority day centres or hostels, home helps or meals on wheels, either in the 6 months before or during the study period. However, two patients in each group reported seeing a social worker during the study period. The two patients in the CPN condition had a total of 22 sessions and the two patients in the GP condition had a total of 14 sessions. Calculations were made on the basis of 1 hour per session.

Social Security payments

As Table 2.3 shows, reported Social Security payments were much the same for each group (with 11 patients in the CPN condition and 12 patients in the GP condition). There were no significant differences over time.

Patients' and relatives' work lost and travel expenses

Travel costs for the two groups were very similar. The figures given relate to cost of bus/train fares or car mileage to travel to the surgery for consultations and/or CPN sessions.

Regarding relatives' loss of work time, one patient in the CPN condition reported that a relative lost a job because of having to take time off to look after her. Seven patients in the CPN condition reported that their relatives sustained a total loss of income due to the problem of £1650 (mean £235.70) while six patients in the GP condition reported that their relatives sustained a total loss of income due to the problem of £850 (mean £141.70).

Patients' other expenses

In the 6 months before the study, three patients in each condition received private outpatient treatment for their problem (Table 2.3).

During the 6 months of the study five patients in each condition received private outpatient treatment for their problem, at a total cost of £910 for the GP group and £715 for the CPN group.

One other patient in the CPN condition reported needing to have a childminder (because of her partial inability to look after her child) at a cost of £50 per week for 12 weeks (total cost £600).

The numbers involved in this data subset were too small to do any analyses. No private inpatient treatment was reported for either group.

Net cost of CPN and GP groups

Table 2.4 shows the net costs for both groups. As indicated above the difference in work absences demonstrates a clear and substantial net benefit associated with CPN treatment. However the table shows no other significant differences between the groups.

DISCUSSION

The implications of the main outcome study are discussed in detail elsewhere (Gournay and Brooking, 1992, 1994). Our economic data covered a very wide range of categories. However, as our results show, much of these data were for a relatively small number of CPNs in two health authorities and for relatively small groups of patients. For example, the use of other psychiatric treatment resources involved six patients only, while only four patients saw a social worker in addition. Therefore, there is of course a possibility that the results from this study may not be representative of the work of CPNs in this area.

Regarding absences from work, patients in the CPN condition had significantly fewer absences from work in the 24 weeks after initial asessment compared with the previous 24 weeks. This reduction was spread over a number of patients rather than being accounted for by one or two individuals. This is the only area in the study (including clinical outcome) where the CPN condition shows any advantage over the GP condition. As Table 2.4 shows, this superiority of the CPN condition at 6 months indicates clear cost reduction to the community in general. However there is no cost reduction to the health care system *per se*. For example, the usage of GP resources (Table 2.5) is much the same for both groups, indicating that referral to the CPN does not save GP time. Indeed, if one considers health care costs alone, patients in the CPN condition are more expensive to treat because of the addition of the CPN to other services.

There are two particular problems connected with our evaluation that do not apply to the economic evaluations of nurse therapy referred to above. First, as O'Donnell, Maynard and Wright (1988) pointed out, nurse therapists were used as substitutes for psychiatric specialists, providing very specific care for a defined group. This is not the case for CPNs in primary health care, as the patient population is arguably more amorphous in character and would probably not have received specialist psychiatric treatment had it not been for the CPN attachment to their primary health care centre. The second problem is far more complex, as it involves the comparative costs of the CPN in this area rather than in any other area of CPN function (for example with long-term serious mental illness). At present, there are no data, other than that of the Springfield Research Team (Paykel and Griffith, 1983; Mangen *et al.*, 1983) that give any indication of CPN cost effectiveness and, as the Springfield study was conducted more than a decade ago, their results have limited contemporary value. From the data gathered in our study, the cost per QALY of CPN treatment can be computed using revised values for the Rosser Matrix obtained from a large random sample of the general population (Gudex *et al.*, 1993) (Table 2.6). Preventing absence from work is worth about 0.1 QALY per year (Disability State 5 versus Disability State 4); 4 days represents 0.0017 of a QALY and the cost per QALY of CPN treatment is £28 000. Of treatments for which cost per QALY are available, we do know that this is at the higher cost end. Although the Wilkinson *et al.* study (1990) was uncontrolled and the cost per QALY was based on older figures than

Table 2.6 'Rosser Matrix' quality adjusted life-years

Disability states	Distress states			
	a	*b*	*c*	*d*
1	(1.00)	0.90	0.85	0.55
2	0.90	0.70	0.60	0.45
3	0.65	0.55	0.50	0.35
4	0.60	0.50	0.45	0.30
5	0.50	0.40	0.35	0.20
6	0.40	0.35	0.30	0.15
7	0.30	0.25	0.20	0.10
8	0.00	0.00	0.00	0.00

we report here, these authors showed that costs per QALY were lower for treating people with schizophrenia than for people with either affective or neurotic disorders (£6000 per QALY for people with schizophrenia, £10 000 for those with an affective disorder and £25 000 for people with neuroses). Therefore it is important, when considering where CPNs might best be utilized, that we have studies of CPN intervention in various settings that include the use of costs per unit of health gain. However, if CPNs are to be relocated, it is difficult to see how one could calculate the economic and human cost of moving CPNs from one area to another and in effect depriving another population of care. White's (1991) data show that currently this deprivation (which has been the result of the move of CPNs to work with less serious mental health problems in primary care) may involve the very vulnerable group of people with chronic schizophrenia who appear less and less on CPN caseloads.

As White (1991) also shows, CPN services are constantly expanding into new areas and focusing on new problem categories. In a sense, therefore, CPNs are now targeting patients who would not previously have sought treatment for their condition. This seems particularly the case in the primary care area. Therefore, this expansion of CPN work (not generally supported by research evidence) may not only leave the very vulnerable population of people with serious mental illness, referred to above, high and dry but may also add considerably to service costs without any real return.

In summary, therefore, our study shows only one significant difference on our economic measures – the reduced absence from work of patients in the CPN condition. This difference results in a substantial net benefit associated with CPN treatment. Although this difference is not mirrored in the clinical outcome measures, it is, as pointed out above, substantial and the reduction in work absence derives from several patients rather than from one or two individuals. In view of the fact that we have very little contemporary evidence of the effectiveness of CPN intervention, this result needs to be considered seriously and helps emphasize the importance of further research in this area.

ACKNOWLEDGEMENTS

We wish to thank Mr Robert Anderson of the Department of Health who gave us considerable helpful assistance in both the planning of the study and the writing of our final report.

We were assisted on the project by Grant Devilly, Louise Geldart, Pam McCarthy, Ann Thomas and Michael Baker. Michael Baker was particularly involved in the design and planning of the economic analysis. We would also like to thank Dr Claire Gudex (Centre for Health Economics, University of York) for very helpful comments on this manuscript and the advisory group who assisted us during our study (this group included Isaac Marks, David Winter, Kate Wooff, John Tait, Veronica Bishop and Tony McDaid). The Department of Health funded the study.

REFERENCES

Brooker, C. and Brown, M. (1986) National follow up survey of practicing nurse therapists, in *Psychiatric Nursing Research*, (ed. J. Brooking), John Wiley, Chichester.

Culyer, A.J. and Wagstaff, A. (1992) *QALYs versus HYEs: A Theoretical Exposition*, Discussion paper 99, Centre for Health Economics, University of York, York.

Gafni, A. (1989) The quality of QALYs: do QALYs measure what they intend to measure? *Health Policy*, **13**, 81–3.

Ginsberg, G. and Marks, I.M. (1977) Costs and benefits of behavioural psychotherapy: a pilot study of neurotics treated by nurse therapists. *Psychological Medicine*, **7**, 685–700.

Ginsberg, G., Marks, I. and Waters, H. (1984) Cost benefit in a controlled trial of nurse therapy for neuroses in primary care. *Psychological Medicine*, **14**, 683–90.

Gournay, K.J.M. and Brooking, J.I. (1992) The CPN in primary care, Report to Department of Health.

Gournay, K.J.M. and Brooking, J.I. (1994) The community psychiatric nurse in primary health care – an outcome study. *British Journal of Psychiatry*, in press.

Gournay, K.J.M., Devilly, G. and Brooker, C. (1993) The CPN in primary care: a pilot study of the process of assessment, in *Community Psychiatric Nursing: A Research Perspective*, vol. 2, (eds C. Brooker and E. White), Chapman & Hall, London.

Gournay, K.J.M. and Newell, R. (1993) *A National Follow-up of Nurse Behaviour Therapists*. Middlesex University Health Research Centre, London

Gudex, C., Kind, P., van Dalen, H. *et al*. (1993) *Compelling Scaling Methods for Health State Valuations – Rosser Revisited*. Centre for Health Economics, University of York, York.

Illing, J., Drinkwater, C., Rogerson, T. *et al*. (1990) Evaluation of community psychiatric nurses in general practice, in *Community Psychiatric Nursing*, (ed. C. Brooker), Chapman & Hall, London.

Knapp, M., Beecham, J., Anderson, J. *et al*. (1990) The TAPS project 3: predicting the costs of closing psychiatric hospitals. *British Journal of Psychiatry*, **157**, 661–70.

Leff, J. (1993) The TAPS project: evaluating community placement of long stay psychiatric placements. *British Journal of Psychiatry*, **162**(Suppl.).

Mangen, S.P., Paykel, E.S., Griffith, J.H. *et al*. (1983) Cost-effectiveness of community psychiatric nurse or out-patient psychiatrist care of neurotic patients. *Psychological Medicine*, **33**, 407–16.

Marks, I.M. (1985) *Psychiatric Nurse Therapists in Primary Care*, RCM Publications, London.

Mehrez, A. and Gafni, A. (1989) Quality Adjusted Life Years, utility, theory and health year equivalents. *Medical Decision Making*, **9**, 142–9.

Muijen, M., Marks, I. and Connolly, J. (1992) Home based care and standard hospital care for patients with severe mental illness. *British Medical Journal*, **304**, 749–54.

O'Donnell, O., Maynard, A. and Wright, K. (1988) *The Economic Evaluation of Mental Health Care: a Review*, Centre for Health Economics Consortium, University of York, York.

Paykel, E.S. and Griffith, J.H. (1983) *Community Psychiatric Nursing for Neurotic Patients*, RCN Publications, London.

Rosser, R.M. and Kind, P. (1978) A scale of valuation of states of illness: is there a social consensus? *International Journal of Epidemiology*, **7**, 347–57.

Rosser, R.M. and Watts, C. (1972) The measurement of hospital output. *International Journal of Epidemiology*, **1**, 361–8.

White, E. (1991) *Third Quinquennial Study of Community Psychiatric Nursing*. University of Manchester, Department of Nursing Studies.

Wilkinson, G., Croft-Jeffreys, C., Krekorianh Mclees, S. and Falloon, I. (1990) QALYs in psychiatric care. *Psychiatric Bulletin*, **14**, 582–5.

CHAPTER THREE

Evaluation of the Tameside Nursing Development Unit for psychosocial interventions

Ian Baguley

INTRODUCTION

This chapter will decribe how, over a period of 3 years, professionals from one health district (Tameside) will be trained in the use of psychosocial intervention techniques and how this work will be evaluated.

The work described in this chapter is happening at a time when a number of initiatives are beginning to make their presence felt. The continuing rundown of psychiatric inpatient beds and the government plans for care in the community (Department of Health, 1989) have placed an intense burden on both families and communities. It is important, therefore, that service responses to these initiatives is coordinated, structured and focused. Serious mental illness, especially schizophrenia, has provided mental health workers with their biggest challenge. Community psychiatric nurses (CPNs), in particular, are subject to a number of pressures that make the organization of their work and the prioritization of referrals difficult. The response of some health authorities and trust boards to the demands of GP fundholders and the requirements of the Care Programme Approach has placed CPNs in an invidious position (CPNA, 1993). While there is evidence that CPNs have moved away from those clients who suffer from a serious mental illness (White, 1990), any efforts made by CPNs to resume effective work with this client group has been made difficult by a lack of clear service direction (Woof, 1992). As Birchwood and Tarrier (1992) point out, unless there is a clear commitment from service managers to facilitate new working practices, the vested interest of established practice will take precedence.

Research carried out over the past 35 years or so clearly demonstrates the effectiveness of using an integrated approach to the care of those patients suffering from a serious mental illness (Brown *et al.*, 1962; Brown, Birley and Wing, 1972; Vaughn and Leff, 1976). The notion of 'expressed emotion' (EE), the development of a stress vulnerability model and the refinement of cognitive behavioural approaches in the treatment of serious mental illness have all contributed to the development of research-based psychosocial intervention techniques. Although most of the work in this area has been restricted to fairly tightly controlled research studies (Leff *et al.*, 1985; Falloon *et al.*, 1985; Hogarty *et al.*, 1986) the work of Brooker and Butterworth (1993) strongly suggests that CPNs can be trained in the effective use of psychosocial intervention techniques.

The incidence of serious mental illness such as schizophrenia has changed little over time and, despite the absence of rigorous diagnostic criteria, has continued to be of the order 0.5–1.0% (Barrowclough and Tarrier, 1992). The implications of these figures for Tameside Health Authority are that between 1250 and 2500 people will develop, or will be suffering from, schizophrenia. As a result of the long-term nature of the illness, prevalence is greater than incidence. Thus the economic cost to the Health Authority (of schizophrenia per case) is likely to be greater than a serious physical illness such as coronary heart disease (Birchwood, Hallett and Preston, 1988).

Traditionally, the treatment of schizophrenia has consisted of the administration of regular neuroleptic medication and admission to hospital at times of crisis. Although CPN services were set up originally to cater for patients recently discharged from hospital, notably those suffering from serious mental illness, there is recent evidence that less time is now spent with this client group than any other (White, 1990; Woof, Goldberg and Fryers, 1988). The growth of 'depot clinics', a central point where patients can go to receive their medication, has not assisted the provision of a personal service able to be responsive to the needs of clients (Turner, 1993). The importance of medication to help clients control distressing symptoms cannot be underestimated, but it is also important that professionals view medication as but one part of a package of care.

BACKGROUND

Tameside Health District provides health care to a population of approximately 250 000 people. The catchment area ranges from Denton in Greater Manchester to Glossop in Derbyshire – a mixture of urban developments and village communities. Mental health care is provided by three multidisciplinary community mental health teams (CMHTs), one based in each locality, three community rehabilitation teams (CRTs) and a district drugs and alcohol service. In addition there is also a community team for people over 65 years old that also provides a service for clients with dementia within each sector. Inpatient facilities are provided by Tameside and Glossop District General Hospital at Ashton-under-Lyne. There are a total of 70 inpatient beds and a psychiatric day hospital on this site. Day facilities are also being developed in each locality.

The community rehabilitation service grew out of a recognition among managers that services for those clients with a serious mental illness required a more flexible service. Previously, specialist rehabilitation services were based around an inpatient ward. Those people living in the community were catered for by the community mental health teams. These teams came under increasing pressure from primary health care referrals and managers recognized that, if people suffering from a serious mental illness were to receive a service that was able to meet their needs such a service needed to be developed and staffed from outside the community mental health teams. In the mid 1980s, a decision was made locally to close the rehabilitation ward and to house clients in supported accommodation in the community. The staff who previously worked on the ward staffed the supported accommodation. As accommodation was found for individual patients, the staff became involved in home visits. Over time, more group homes were established with the cooperation of local housing associations and staff were recruited to work in the community. Each CRT now consists of support workers and 'F'-graded CPNs and each team is managed by a 'G'-grade CPN. The rehabilitation service, including group homes, is managed by an 'H'-grade manager.

In 1992, two important developments occurred. Firstly, the Care Programme Approach (Department of Health, 1990a) was introduced and those clients suffering from serious mental illness that were cared for by the CMHTs began to be transferred to the CRT. So far 270 clients have been transferred to the CRT and the transfer has continued as more resources are put in place. Secondly, Tameside Mental Health Services successfully applied for Kings Fund nursing development moneys in order to employ a worker who would facilitate the development of psychosocial intervention techniques within the district. Both of these developments have demonstrated Tameside's commitment to prioritizing services for patients with a serious mental illness. The assessments devised for the Care Programme Approach are both thorough and structured and have been designed specifically to ensure that the service is driven by patient need.

DEMOGRAPHIC PROFILE

All demographic and assessment data relating to Tameside Health District has been collected by the community rehabilitation team through the Care Programme Approach Support System (Tameside and Glossop Mental Health

Services, 1992). A total of 270 clients receive a service from the community rehabilitation team (Table 3.1), 148 male and 122 female. Although most clients are single (166), the majority live with a close relative (127); 41 live in shared accommodation and five live with a friend; 77 clients live alone. Most clients live in rented accommodation (162) and 63 own their own homes. One person is of no fixed address. Only two clients are in full time employment, eight are in sheltered employment; 216 clients are either unemployed (45) or registered as long-term sick (171). The vast majority of clients have a diagnosis of schizophrenia (194) or affective psychosis (41) (Table 3.1).

Table 3.1 Diagnosis of patients served by the community rehabilitation team ($n = 270$)

Schizophrenia	194
Affective psychosis	41
Depression	10
Other psychosis	8
Not known	5
Neurotic disorder	3
Non-specific mental illness	3
Personality problems	2
Learning difficulties	1
Organic psychosis	1
Missing cases	2

ASSESSMENT DATA

The assessment of patients focuses upon 12 areas: caring network, social network, emotional support, medication, symptoms, employment/vocation, self-care, housekeeping, accommodation, finance, physical health and safety. Problem severity is self-assessed on a six-point Likert scale, a score of 0 indicating no problem, 5 the most severe problems. 'Good' and 'average' indicate no or slight problem, not significant. All other scores indicate a problem that has a significant effect on the client and therefore requires focused intervention. Problems are recorded at initial assessment and again at review or discharge (Table 3.2). Reviews are carried out at no more than 6-monthly intervals.

Detailed analysis of these data will be reported elsewhere. However, for the purposes of this chapter the data have been separated into two main areas: those scores that indicate significant distress for the client (slight–extreme) and those that do not (good–average). The mean scores for the total population ($n = 260$) are also given. 'Caring network' covers the client's relationships with carers (a score of 0 represents full support from the carers) without

Table 3.2 Problem/severity matrix ($n = 270$)

Problem	Severity		
	Good/average (0–1)	Slight–extreme (2–5)	Mean score (0–5)
Caring network	131	129	1.50
Social network	78	182	2.16
Emotional support	73	187	1.93
Medication	136	124	1.49
Symptoms	102	158	1.82
Employment	135	125	1.69
Self-care	135	125	1.48
Housekeeping	117	143	1.60
Accommodation	198	62	0.87
Finance	161	99	1.22
Physical health	187	73	1.04
Safety	189	71	1.00
Missing cases = 10			

being intrusive. The carers' understanding of the client's problem is excellent. Any score other than 0 indicates the need for more focused clinical work. A score of 1 indicates self-regulating, minor tensions, irritations or crisis that do not persist. A score of 2 indicates problems that, while still of a minor nature, are more long-term and persistent sources of stress. Scores of 3, 4 or 5 indicate increasing amounts of conflict and distress between the client and the carer. Although 64 clients scored 0 at initial assessment and 67 scored 1, the scores of 129 clients indicate a need for more intensive family work. The mean score at initial assessment for this area was 1.5.

'Social network' is designed to cover social functioning, friendships and interpersonal relationships. The mean score in this area at initial assessment was 2.16. A total of 78 clients scored 0 or 1, indicating either a good social life with no reliance on institutional activities or participation in some non-stigmatizing social activity; 182 clients scored higher, indicating that developing social relationships is a major problem for most clients. The category of 'emotional support' aims to provide an indication of the ability of clients to seek their own support at times of crisis and upset. The mean score for this area at first assessment was 1.93; 73 clients scored 0 or 1 while 187 clients scored 2 or higher, which indicated that most clients have little in the way of independent emotional support or are unable to use the support available and, consequently, rely on the helping agencies. For the category of 'medication' 136 clients are reported taking medication freely with few or no side effects, or did not require medication; ,

124 clients experienced problems, ranging from persisting difficulties with side effects to more severe side effects. The mean score for this area is 1.49.

The mean score for 'symptoms' is 1.82. A total of 102 clients did not experience symptoms that were serious enough to disrupt their social functioning or their intellectual ability, while 158 clients experienced symptoms ranging from mild symptoms through to severe symptoms that disrupt their life completely and make communication impossible. In the 'employment' section, although most clients were either unemployed or in receipt of long-term sickness benefit, 135 clients were reportedly satisfied with their daily activities (mean 1.69), while 125 clients were dissatisfied. A mean score of 1.48 was recorded on the 'self-care' problem matrix: 135 people had no problems in this area or were able to ask for assistance when required, while 125 people needed varying degrees of help in achieving daily living tasks such as shopping or cooking or personal hygiene.

In the 'accommodation' category, 198 clients lived in accommodation that was either adequate or only a source of minor problems; 62 clients experienced more serious problems. A total of 161 clients had few or no financial problems; 99 clients experienced more worrying financial problems; of these 17 were in the severe to extreme range and would be a source of major stress. On the 'physical health' matrix, clients enjoyed good to average physical health, 66 clients experienced slight to moderate problems, and seven experienced severe or extreme physical problems. 'Safety' covers personal safety – clients who might be at risk from others; history of violence towards others; history of criminal activity; household insecure, etc. On this matrix 189 clients were thought to be 'safe' or at only minimum risk; 71 clients were felt to be vulnerable in some way.

These data indicate that a substantial number of clients experience problems that are likely to have a detrimental effect on the course of their illness. In addition, these problems cover a broad spectrum from interpersonal difficulties to personal safety, from financial and housing difficulties to persisting symptoms and medication problems. Such a range of problems demands a well coordinated service that is able to prioritize work and evaluate its effectiveness. It is known that the community rehabilitation team is in regular contact with 270 clients, and that a substantial number of these clients experience persistent problems that impact directly and regularly on their illness. It is also suspected that a further 230 clients who suffer from a serious mental illness were waiting to be referred to the CRT. There is no information readily available about the needs of these clients. The need to prioritize cases that the CRT were already working with was essential if this service is to continue to be effective. The utilization of measures to collect data related to outcome, which will measure the effect that interventions are having on clients and carers, will be an invaluable aid to this process.

EDUCATION

People with a serious mental illness have been identified as a service priority (Department of Health, 1990a, 1992; Butterworth, 1993). The effectiveness of training nurses with the specialist skills required to work effectively with this client group has been demonstrated (Brooker, Barrowclough and Tarrier, 1992; Brooker *et al.*, 1993). The desire for interdisciplinary, skills-based training is set out in Working Paper 10 (Department of Health, 1990b).

A skills-based training course in psychosocial intervention techniques has been set up in Tameside, based on a problem-centred approach to people with serious mental illness and their families. The course is multidisciplinary and aims to encourage teamwork and understanding. Previous courses focused on this area, most notably those run by the University of Manchester and Sheffield Hallam University, produced practitioners who were skilled, enthusiastic and highly motivated. Unfortunately, when these workers returned to their places of work, they were often isolated and marginalized. Consequently, the return of the 'Hero Innovator' became a reality (Georgiades and Phillimore, 1975).

An effective way to address this problem might be to train a team or a group of workers from across the whole range of mental health services within a health district. To this end nurses who work on the inpatient unit, day services, rehabilitation team and primary-health-care-based community services, along with workers from care of the elderly service, attend the Tameside course. Birchwood and Tarrier (1992) emphasize the importance of a management framework to enable this kind of work and argue that without the management will, the vested interests of established practice will continue to take priority.

There is evidence that nurses who undergo formal training in psychosocial intervention offer a more effective service to clients than those nurses who have not undergone such training (Brooker and Butterworth, 1993). A training programme has been established for staff from across the mental health services within Tameside Health District. Although most of the staff who attend this course are from the rehabilitation team, there are also staff from the inpatient unit, day services and primary-health-based services. The course is being taught by the present writer and two CPNs who have had previous training in psychosocial intervention. The training aims to give students a broad introduction to the theory that underpins psychosocial intervention and an opportunity to acquire and practise skills under close, clinical supervision. The skills module focuses primarily on engagement and assessment, followed by an introduction to interventions. The course content is presented within the framework of a stress vulnerability model of illness (Zubin and Spring, 1977). Assessment is emphasized as the cornerstone of future interventions with a client and his or her family. Thorough assessment provides a number of useful functions: firstly it gives an opportunity for the client and family to tell their 'stories', often for the first time; secondly, it gives the nurse a valuable insight into the problems experienced by clients and families; and finally, it allows the collection of baseline data with which to measure change. Students on this course are encouraged to form a therapeutic alliance with families and carers and to acknowledge the families and clients as experts in coping with what is often a difficult situation (Kuipers, Leff and Lam, 1992; Barrowclough and Tarrier, 1992; Falloon *et al.*, 1993). The process of assessment will help to identify the strengths and needs of individual family members, facilitating more focused interventions. All structured assessment tools have been chosen because they have both a clinical and research utility.

It has long been recognized that patients who suffered from schizophrenia experienced severe impairments in both social and personal functioning (Kraepelin, 1919; Falloon, Boyd and McGill, 1984; Birchwood, Hallett and Preston, 1988). Social and personal functioning is now accepted as an important indicator of outcome in patients suffering from schizophrenia (Mauser and Sayers, 1992). The Social Functioning Scale and the Personal Functioning Scale will be used to collect baseline data (Birchwood *et al.*, 1990); both measures will be repeated at regular intervals in order to provide an indication of change.

Previous research and interventions have generally focused on the effects of the family on the client. There is now a substantial body of evidence that shows that family members themselves experience a range of problems through having to care for an ill relative at home (Schultz, House and Andrews, 1986; Orford, 1987; Hatfield, 1987; Halford, 1992). The General Health Questionnaire (Goldberg, 1972; Goldberg and Hillier, 1978) will be used to measure the amount of minor psychiatric morbidity experienced by family members.

When caring for a relative who suffers from a long-term serious mental illness, family members often experience a degree of burden that substantially effects their quality of life (Wallace, 1985; Newton, 1988). The Lancashire Quality of Life Profile (Oliver, 1991) will be used to collect data and measure change.

Educating families about the illness their relative suffers from has been a major part of a number of intervention studies (Lam, 1993). Despite this, the explicit function of education is uncertain (Barrowclough and Tarrier, 1992). However, if clients and families are to understand their experiences, they need to be given information about the illness (Falloon *et al.*, 1993). Hatfield (1990) reports that relatives constantly request information both about the illness and advice on coping strategies. Barrowclough *et al.* (1987) assert that, if professionals are going to give information to relatives, they should be assured that the relatives have fully understood what they have said. Professionals should not assume that relatives automatically understand. The Knowledge About Schizophrenia Interview (KASI) is a semi-structured interview that aims to elicit a relative's functional knowledge about the illness and provides information that enables an education package to be built on the strengths of the relative and target knowledge deficits (Barrowclough *et al.*, 1987).

Traditionally, the assessment of the symptoms of the illness has been a matter for the medical profession. Other professions, such as nursing, often without any formal training in the assessment of symptoms, have been encouraged to report their observations to doctors. Nurses undergoing psychosocial intervention training are now being taught how to assess symptoms by using the Manchester or K-G-V scale (Krawiecka, Goldberg and Vaughan 1977). This scale rates nine areas based on observation and interview and examines both positive and negative symptoms. One of the additional benefits of using such a scale is that the use of a common language between professions facilitates teamwork. Although all the data from these assessment measures will be collected at 6-monthly intervals for research and evaluation purposes, staff will be encouraged to use them more regularly where appropriate.

There seems to be a genuine attempt by central government to encourage health authorities to focus resources on patients who suffer from serious mental illness. Tameside Health Authority, in order to keep up the momentum of a rapidly changing and innovative rehabilitation service, successfully applied for Kings Fund moneys to employ a project worker whose sole aim was to facilitate the development of psychosocial intervention techniques for people with a serious mental illness.

ACKNOWLEDGEMENTS

The writer is indebted to Len Bowers from Tameside Training and Development Association and Paul Roe from Tameside Social Services for giving access to data from the Tameside Care Programme Support System.

REFERENCES

Barrowclough, C. and Tarrier, N. (1992) *Families of Schizophrenic Patients: Cognitive Behavioural Interventions*, Chapman & Hall, London.

Barrowclough, C., Tarrier, N., Watts, S. *et al.* (1987) Assessing the functional value of relatives' reported knowledge about schizophrenia. *British Journal of Psychiatry*, **151**, 1–8.

Birchwood, M., Hallett, S. and Preston, M. (1988) *Schizophrenia: An Integrated Approach To Research and Treatment*, Longman, Harlow.

Birchwood, M., Smith, J., Cochrane, R. *et al.* (1990) The Social Functioning Scale: the development and validation of a scale of social adjustment for use in family intervention programmes with schizophrenic patients. *British Journal of Psychiatry*, **157**, 853–9.

Birchwood, M. and Tarrier, N. (1992) *Innovations in the Psychological Management of Schizophrenia: Assessment, Treatment and Services*, John Wiley, Chichester.

Brooker, C., Barrowclough, C. and Tarrier, N. (1992) Training community psychiatric nurses in psychosocial interventions: evaluating the impact of health education for relatives. *Journal of Clinical Nursing*, **1**, 19–25.

Brooker, C. and Butterworth, T. (1993) Training in psychosocial intervention: the impact on the role of community psychiatric nurses. *Journal of Advanced Nursing*, **18**, 583–90.

Brooker, C., Tarrier, N., Barrowclough, C. *et al.*, (1993) Skills for CPNs working with seriously mentally ill people: the outcome of a trial of psychosocial intervention, in *Community Psychiatric Nursing: A Research Perspective*, vol. 2, (eds C. Brooker and E. White) Chapman & Hall, London.

Brown, G.W., Birley, J.L.T. and Wing, J.K. (1972) Influence of family life on the course of schizophrenic disorders: a replication. *British Journal of Psychiatry*, **121**, 241–58.

Brown, G.W., Monck, E.M., Carstairs, G.M. and Wing, J.K. (1962) Influence of family life on the course of schizophrenic illness. *British Journal of Preventive and Social Medicine*, **16**, 55–68.

Butterworth C.A.B, (1993) Paper presented to a meeting of representatives of seconding health districts to the Thorn Nurse Initiative. Department of Nursing, University of Manchester, Manchester.

CPNA (1993) A call for action: the CPNA response to the 1993 Mental health nursing review. *Community Psychiatric Nursing Journal*, **13**, 32–8.

Department of Health (1989) *Caring for People*, HMSO, London.

Department of Health (1990a) *The Care Programme Approach for People with a Mental Illness Referred to the Specialist Psychiatric Services*, HMSO, London.

Department of Health (1990b) *Education and Training, Working Paper 10*, Department of Health, London.

Department of Health (1992) *Clinical Standards Advisory Group*, Department of Health, London.

Falloon, I.R.H., Boyd, J.L. and McGill, C.W. (1984) *Family Care of Schizophrenia*, Guilford Press, New York.

Falloon, I.R.H., Boyd, J.L. and McGill, C.W. *et al.* (1985) Family management in the prevention of morbidity of schizophrenia: Clinical outcome of a two year longitudinal study. *Archives of General Psychiatry*, **42**, 887–96.

Falloon, I.R.H., Lapporta, M., Fadden, G. and Graham-Hole, V. (1993) *Managing Stress in Families: Cognitive Behavioural Strategies for Enhancing Coping Skills*, Routledge, London.

Georgiades, N.J. and Phillimore, L. (1975) The myth of the hero-innovator and alternative strategies for organizational change, in *Behaviour Modification with the Severely Retarded*, (eds C.C. Kiernan and F.P. Woodford), Associated Scientific, New York.

Goldberg, D.P. (1972) *The Detection of Psychiatric Illness by Questionnaire*, Maudsley Monographs, Oxford University Press, London.

Goldberg, D.P. and Hillier, V. (1978) A scaled version of the General Health Questionnaire. *Psychological Medicine*, **9**, 139–46.

Halford, W.K. (1992) Assessment of family interaction with a schizophenic member, in *Schizophrenia: An Overview and Practical Handbook*, (ed. D.J. Kavanagh), Chapman & Hall, London.

Hatfield, A. (1987) Social support and family coping, in *Families of the Mentally Ill: Coping and Adaptation*, (eds A. Hatfield and H.P. Lefley), Guilford Press, New York.

Hatfield, A. (1990) *Family Education in Mental Illness*, Guilford Press, New York.

Hogarty, G., Anderson, C.M., Reiss, D.J. *et al.* (1986) Family psychoeducation, social skills training and maintenance chemotherapy in the aftercare treatment of schizophrenia. 1: One-year effects of a controlled study on relapse and expressed emotion. *Archives of General Psychiatry*, **43**, 633–42.

Kraepelin, D.E. (1919) *Dementia Praecox and Paraphrenia*, (trans. R.M. Barclay), E. & S. Livingstone, Edinburgh.

Krawieka, M., Goldberg, D. and Vaughan, M. (1977) A standardised psychiatric assessment scale for chronic psychotic patients. *Acta Psychiatrica Scandinavica*, **55**, 299–308.

Kuipers, L., Leff, J. and Lam, D. (1992) *Family Work for Schizophrenia: A Practical Guide*, Gaskell, Royal College of Psychiatrists, London.

Lam, D. (1991) Psychosocial intervention: a review of empirical studies. *Psychological Medicine*, **21**, 423–41.

Leff, J.P., Kuipers, L., Berkowitz, R. and Sturgeon, D. (1985) A controlled trial of social intervention in the families of schizophrenic patients: two year follow up. *British Journal of Psychiatry*, **146**, 594–600.

Mauser, K.T. and Sayers, M.S.D. (1992) Social skills assessment, in *Schizophrenia: An Overview and Practical Handbook*, (ed. D.J. Kavanagh), Chapman & Hall, London.

Newton, J. (1988) *Preventing Mental Illness*, Routledge, London.

Oliver, J.P.J. (1991) The social care directive: development of a quality of life profile for use in community services for the mentally ill. *Social Work and Social Sciences Review*, **3**, 5–45.

Orford, J. (1987) *Coping with Disorder in the Family*, Croom Helm, Beckenham.

Schultz, S.C., House, L. and Andrews, M.B. (1986) *Helping Families in a Schizophrenia Programme*, American Psychiatric Press, New York.

Tameside and Glossop Mental Health Service (1992) *The Care Programme Approach Support System*, Tameside and Glossop Mental Health Service, Ashton-under-Lyne.

Turner, G. (1993) Client/CPN contact during the administration of depot medications: implication for practice, in *Community Psychiatric Nursing: A Research Perspective*, (eds C. Brooker and E. White), Chapman & Hall, London.

Vaughn, C.E. and Leff, J.P. (1976) The influence of family and social factors on the course of psychiatric illness. *British Journal of Psychiatry*, **129**, 125–37.

Wallace, M. (1985) When freedom is a life sentence. *The Times*, **16 Dec**.

White, E. (1990) *The Third Quinquennial National Community Psychiatric Nursing Survey*, Department of Nursing, University of Manchester, Manchester.

Woof, K. (1992) Service organisation and planning, in *Innovations in the Psychological*

Management of Schizophrenia: Assessment, Treatment and Services, (eds M. Birchwood and N. Tarrier), John Wiley, Chichester.

Woof, K., Goldberg, D.P. and Fryers, T. (1988) The practice of community psychiatric nursing and mental health social work in Salford: some implications for community care. *British Journal of Psychiatry*, **152**, 783–92.

Zubin, J. and Spring, B. (1977) Vulnerability: a new view of schizophrenia. *Journal of Abnormal Psychology*, **86**, 260–6.

CHAPTER FOUR

Normalizing psychiatry: the professionalization of community psychiatric nursing in the UK and Italy

Monica Savio

This chapter presents a summary of findings from a comparative research study on British and Italian community psychiatric nursing. The aim is twofold. First to analyse similarities and differences between CPNs' practice and professional experience in the two countries. This is linked with the historical and cultural developments of community care in the UK and Italy. The context in which community psychiatric nursing emerged and developed is fundamental to understanding the experience of British and Italian CPNs. Secondly the chapter aims at raising attention on a topical issue for the future of community psychiatric nursing. This is the analysis of the opportunities for the specialty to undertake further professionalization. At a stage at which new approaches in psychiatric care call for the normalization of clients' lives, it is necessary to see how professional practices can be normalizing, and whether this can be directed towards professionalization. The questions to be answered are therefore: (1) What does professionalization mean, i.e. does it necessarily mean specialization? and (2) What is the role of community psychiatric nursing in the transition from hospital- to community-based practices?

The different CPNs' experiences in Britain and Italy suggest interesting aspects of the understanding of professional issues crossnationally. Results indicate that in both countries, community psychiatric nursing is in a transitional stage in which possibly the opportunities for new professional developments tend towards an epistemological chasm. Despite the differences between British and Italian practice, some important elements are common to both countries. Among these are (1) that community psychiatric nursing has now little in common with hospital-based psychiatric nursing and (2) that the development of the profession in the community is such as to render CPNs' subordination to, and operational dependence on, the medical hegemony less and less important.

METHODS

Respondents were sampled among community psychiatric nursing teams in the UK and community mental health centres in Italy. Respondents were not randomly sampled among the totality of British and Italian community psychiatric nurses. The analysis which follows is not therefore representative of all CPNs working in the two countries. Investigation was carried out by means of two questionnaires. The first multiple-choice questionnaire aimed at collecting data about nurses' training, community practice, organization and professional identity. Data from the two samples were compared and tested with the chi-square and Mann–Whitney tests whenever appropriate. The second questionnaire focused on the analysis of nurses' ideologies of psychiatric care. Respondents were asked to state their degree of agreement/disagreement with a number of statements on mental illness. The methodology for the elaboration of this questionnaire was derived from Strauss (1964). His research on the relevance of psychiatric ideologies within two large mental hospitals was conducted through the analysis of the degree of professional approval and disapproval concerning specific ideological statements. Results were compared between the two samples and tested using the Mann–Whitney test. The present chapter will focus on a selection of the research findings.

BACKGROUND

An understanding of similarities and differences between British and Italian CPNs is to be linked with the organizational structure which in the two countries characterizes nursing practice in the community. The organization of work – interpreted as the professional hierarchy and the operational structure and planning – is the expression of the cultural, historical and ideological meanings attached to community care in the UK and Italy. Differences between the organization of British and Italian CPNs are the baseline for the anlaysis of the professional experience crossnationally.

CPNs from the British sample are organized in monodisciplinary teams exclusively composed of nurses and hierarchically structured. Two of the teams interviewed were hospital-based, while the third was community-based. However, most of nurses' work is community-oriented; hence nursing practice is prevailingly community-based. This reflects the historical development of community psychiatric nursing in Britain, which parallels strategies of community care implementation at the national level. CPNs were in fact firstly employed in community follow-up programmes during the middle 1950s, when the prevailing care model was hospital-centred. Since then, community care has tended to slowly but progressively replace hospital-based care models. Paralleling such developments CPNs have constantly increased in numbers. In 1954 there were four CPNs, 266 in 1966, 1667 in 1980 and 2758 in 1985. In 1990 the total CPN workforce was estimated to be 4490.

The last CPN survey highlights a distinction between CPNs' main basis and operational basis. For most CPNs the operational basis is the community: only 22.6% of nurses in the UK have their operational basis in a hospital. This points out a trend towards following clients in the community rather than referring them to hospital for community follow-up. Specialization also developed among CPNs. About 42% of nurses specialize in a particular client group, and among these 59.5% specialize in the care of the elderly. In the UK 14% of nurses also specialize in a specific therapeutic approach, of which the most developed are family and behaviour therapy.

Data from the comparative research tend to confirm this trend among the British sample. This seems to show that community psychiatric nursing has changed from a specialized function of hospital care to a pioneer for community care developments. Educational changes within the profession should be analysed according to this key. Specific CPN training began during the 1970s. The establishment of a 36-week course on community psychiatric nursing indicates a need to distinguish between hospital and community competences, although the course is not mandatory and only a minority of CPNs have undertaken it. There are in fact change-blocking factors that do not facilitate the professional transition. Modifications introduced in 1982 in the Registered Mental Nurse training were intended to make nurses more flexibly allocated either to hospital or community work. The syllabus was modified by the introduction of the 'nursing process', which included elements of social policy, psychology and sociology. If on the one hand this might have increased nurses' flexibility, on the other hand it certainly hinders the establishment of a community psychiatric nursing specific professional identity. In part this also reflects the ideology of psychiatric care in Britain, whereby community care is viewed as complementary to hospital care and not yet as its replacement.

The British CPNs interviewed are representative of this transitional stage. From a professional viewpoint they are oriented towards a future as independent practitioners. Operationally, they work within the contradictory hospital/ community dichotomy, which requires them to retain elements of the hospital culture mixed with a community orientation.

The comparison with the Italian situation is quite striking. Italian CPNs are multidisciplinary-based. They operate within community mental health centres (CMHCs) together with psychiatrists, psychologists and social workers.

There is no hierarchy within nursing, but there is a team hierarchical structure in which the consultant psychiatrist carries the main responsibility. This type of organization is common throughout Italy to all nurses in psychiatric care. In some CMHCs, nurses also rotate on ward duty in the district general hospital where a 15-bedded psychiatric ward for every 200 000 of the population is reserved for compulsory admission. However, this is not the case for the CPNs interviewed.

Community psychiatric nursing has, in Italy, a much shorter history than its British counterpart. The first experiences of community psychiatric nursing developed at the end of the 1960s, when community programmes started to be piloted following the French example of *psychiatrie du sector*. The deinstitutionalization movement, which found its major promoter in Dr Franco Basaglia, also emerged during the 1960s and gained increasing importance throughout the 1970s. In 1978 Law 180 (known as the Psychiatric Reform) prescribed the running down of psychiatric hospitals and their replacement with CMHCs. In many parts of Italy, including the regions where the present study was carried out, Law 180 came to legitimize an already established community care policy. The role of nurses was then fundamental, in that they represented the main professional link for patients discharged from hospital and followed up in the community. Then, as now, community care was not regarded as an alternative to hospital care, but as the only feasible option in psychiatric care. The rejection of hospital psychiatry also brought a radical revision of traditional professional competences. Following this, mental health workers, and nurses in particular, undertook *ad hoc* community training based on the needs of the local population. This form of training is still currently the only one available for nurses who wish to work in community psychiatry. Yet it has never been institutionalized so that it does not provide specific qualifications and training contents and methods, as well as its availability, greatly vary all over Italy. In practice the organization of training is delegated to the CMHCs' discretion. Most of the nurses interviewed for this research undertook local training in the CMHCs where they operate.

The difference with the British situation is quite evident. Both in Britain and in Italy, community psychiatric nursing emerged and grew following, and in some instances even anticipating, community care developments. Yet in Britain community care has been generated from within hospital psychiatry; in a sense it is a logical development of a psychiatric epistemology which is still hospital-rooted. As a consequence, nursing training has been modified, but not radically changed. In Italy, on the other hand, community care came into being as a rejection of hospital care and was professional-led rather than government-led, as it mainly is in Britain. It therefore produced an epistemological chasm in psychiatry. According to this approach, nursing training could not be simply modified but it had to be significantly changed. In addition, prior to the reform movement hospital training for psychiatric nursing was also loosely defined and based more on custodial than clinical

Table 4.1 Comparison between British and Italian CPNs' training

Country	Training	Orientation	Qualification	Mandatory
UK	3 years RMN	Predominantly clinical, specific on mental health	Registered Mental Nurse	Yes
	36 weeks CPN	Community-oriented	Community Psychiatric Nurse	No
	ENB courses	Different subjects: social/psychological/clinical	No specific qualification	No: considered to be post-qualification courses
Italy	3 years nursing training	Medical; loose and generic on mental health	*Infermiere professionale* (registered nurse)	Yes: only recently as a requirement to work in community psychiatry
	No training requirement, inservice training	Social, community-oriented	*Operatore psichiatrico* (mental health worker)	Not formally: training is organized by the team according to local needs
	No training requirement, hospital training	Medical; mental-hospital-based	Psychiatric nurses; obsolete qualification available during the asylum years	No: training courses were left to hospital directors' discretion
	Post-qualifying courses equivalent to ENB	Different subjects: social, psychological, medical	No qualification	Not formally

Table 4.2 CPN organization in the UK and in Italy

	UK	Italy
Basis	Community/hospital	Community
Team	CPNs teams	Multidisciplinary teams
Career	Upgrading system	No career opportunities

functions. It was not therefore difficult for nurses to give up their custodial professional identity in order to undertake an ongoing educational process which required of them to be active agents rather than passive executors.

Differences between British and Italian CPN training are indicated in Table 4.1. Table 4.2 illustrates the organization of community psychiatric nursing in the two countries. In contrast to their British colleagues, Italian CPNs do not have specific training in mental health or access to post-qualifying courses for community work. In fact, the qualification of 'psychiatric nurse' does not exist in Italy. This has consequences on the self-perceived professional identity of Italian nurses, who cannot rely on an institutionally acknowledged specialization (RMN/CPN courses in Britain), nor on organizational structures which specifically identify the profession (CPN teams in Britain). On the other hand, the development of community care in Italy is such as to free nurses from hospital boundaries, so that a neat break with the past hospital role has been established.

FINDINGS

The following is a summary of the results from the comparative study of British and Italian CPNs. The selection of data attempts at providing an overall sketch of community psychiatric nursing in the two countries. In particular, information will focus on the professional background of the nurses interviewed, on their clientele, work practices and ideologies of care.

SAMPLES

Interviews have been carried out with 63 nurses in the UK and 56 nurses in Italy. The British sample consists of nurses working in three community psychiatric nursing units. The Italian sample includes nurses working in seven CMHCs, attached to three health districts. Both in the UK and in Italy nearly all the nurses attached to the centres participated in the research. The Italian sample includes the three varieties of nursing qualifications currently present in Italy, i.e. psychiatric nurses trained in the hospital prior to the Psychiatric Reform (30.4%), registered general nurses (46.5%) and psychiatric workers trained in the community (23.2%). All British nurses have had an RMN training and about one-fifth of them also undertook the CPN post-qualifying course (20.3%).

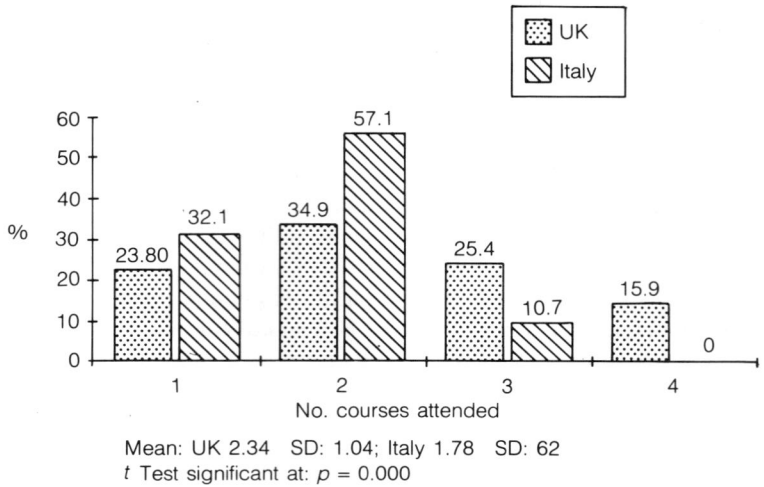

Mean: UK 2.34   SD: 1.04; Italy 1.78   SD: 62
t Test significant at: *p* = 0.000

Figure 4.1 Number of training courses attended in the UK and in Italy.

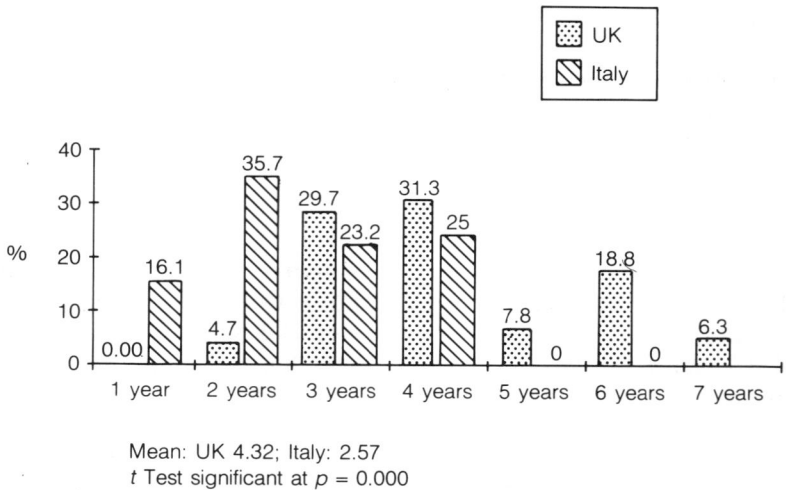

Mean: UK 4.32; Italy: 2.57
t Test significant at *p* = 0.000

Figure 4.2 Period spent training in the UK and in Italy.

TRAINING

Comparatively, Italian nurses have had less professional education than their British colleagues, in terms both of the number of courses attended and of time spent in training. The number of professional courses attended by British nurses is from one to five, and from one to three for Italian nurses. As shown in Figure 4.1, attendance at two professional courses is the modal value both for Britain and for Italy, being the experience of respectively 34.9% and 57.1%. By adding the values for three, four and five courses attended, we can see that 76.2% of British CPNs and 67.8% of the Italians have attended at least two professional courses. In terms of time spent for education, training lasts for a total amount of at least 3 years for 93.9% of British nurses and 48.2% of Italian nurses (Figure 4.2).

Training satisfaction ranks higher among the British sample, where only 14.3% of nurses show little or no satisfaction as to the professional education received, compared to 46.4% of Italian nurses. For both samples the modal position is 'quite satisfied' but, while the majority of British nurses express satisfaction with training, Italian nurses are almost equally split between those who are satisfied and those who are hardly satisfied (Figure 4.3). The comparison between the two sample groups is statistically significant (chi-square $p = 0.000$).

There is a significant difference between nurses attitudes towards the professional education received. The training received is, according to 60.7% of Italian nurses, unsuitable for their present community job, whereas only 25.4% of British nurses found their professional education inadequate to their actual post (chi-square significant at $p = 0.000$). Despite this difference, both Italian and British nurses expressed a strong need to further their professional education (92.9% of Italian nurses and 82.5% of British nurses expressed willingness to do so). Overall the comparison between training practices in the two countries indicates that Italian nurses have been quantitatively and qualitatively less trained than their British colleagues. Specialization in psychiatry occurred for Italian CPNs while already working, mainly in the form of an on-going professional education tailored according to the organizational needs and philosophy of the community centres where they practise. On the one hand, therefore, there is a lack of formal acknowledgement of this form of training, as there is no provision for making it institutionalized and officially recognized. On the other, there is no standardization of community nursing practice and as a consequence nurses enjoy considerable professional autonomy, but also lack means of identification with the profession.

That both British and Italian respondents expressed the need to further their professional education indicates the transitional character of the professional role, as a result of the move from the hospital to the community. Although better trained, British nurses appear to have to modify the hospital-based role internalized during training. Indirectly, this indicates that the shift from hospital to community implies not only a physical move from the place of care, but the need for codifying new intervention models according to the community needs. The development of the present chapter will progressively add elements to support this hypothesis.

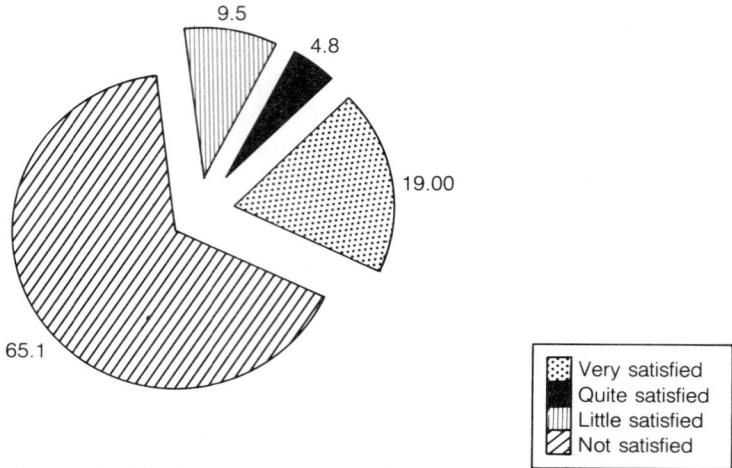

9.5
4.8
19.00
65.1

Very satisfied
Quite satisfied
Little satisfied
Not satisfied

*Among the British sample one respondent did not answer the question, and has not been included in the graphic.
(a)

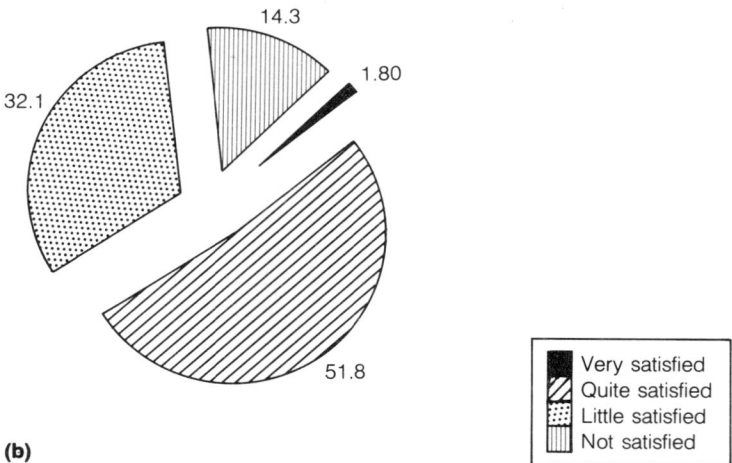

14.3
1.80
32.1
51.8

Very satisfied
Quite satisfied
Little satisfied
Not satisfied

(b)

Figure 4.3 Percentage of nurses satisfied with the training received in **(a)** the UK and **(b)** Italy.

CLIENTELE AND WORK PRACTICES

There is a highly significant difference between the two samples in the comparison between the number of long-term mentally ill clients on nurses' caseloads. All Italian nurses have on their caseload long-term mentally ill clients, and 48 out of 56 have more than half of their caseload made up of this category of client. A total of 11 British nurses do not have long-term mentally ill clients on their caseload, and only 32 out of 63 have more than half of their caseload consisting of this type of client (Table 4.3). Out of 56 Italian CPNs, 46 have more than half of their caseload made up of clients who had a previous hospital admission. This is true only for 32 British CPNs out of 63 (Table 4.4).

Table 4.3 Number of long-term mentally ill clients on nurses' caseload (Mann–Whitney corrected for ties; two-tailed; $p = 0.001$; percentage in parentheses)

No.	UK (n = 63)	Italy (n = 56)
None	11 (17.5)	–
Less than half	20(31.7)	6(10.7)
More than half	12(19.0)	29(51.8)
All of them	20(31.7)	19(33.9)
No answer	–	2 (3.6)

Table 4.4 Number of clients with previous hospital admission on nurses' caseload (Mann–Whitney corrected for ties; two-tailed; $p = 0.007$; percentage in parentheses)

No.	UK (n = 63)	Italy (n = 56)
None	5 (7.8)	–
Less than half	26(41.2)	10(17.9)
More than half	15(24.0)	28(50.0)
All of them	17(27.0)	18(32.1)

The type of clientele in terms of diagnostic category also presents significant differences in the comparison between British and Italian nurses. There are six British CPNs who do not have clients diagnosed with psychosis and 31 who have less than half of their caseload made up of clients diagnosed with psychosis, while all Italian CPNs have in their caseload clients diagnosed

Table 4.5 Number of clients with a medical diagnosis of psychosis on nurses' caseload (Mann–Whitney corrected for ties; two-tailed; $p = 0.000$; percentage in parentheses)

No.	UK (n = 63)	Italy (n = 56)
None	17 (9.5)	0 (0)
Less than half	29(49.2)	6(10.7)
More than half	21(33.3)	38(67.9)
All of them	5 (7.9)	12(21.4)

Table 4.6 Number of clients with a medical diagnosis of neurosis on nurses' caseload (Mann–Whitney corrected for ties; two-tailed; $p = 0.000$; percentage in parentheses)

No.	UK (n = 63)	Italy (n = 56)
None	17(27.0)	28(50.0)
Less than half	29(46.0)	28(50.0)
More than half	14(22.2)	0 (0)
All of them	3 (4.7)	0 (0)

with psychosis, and for the majority of them the caseload consists of this cateogry of client. Conversely, 28 Italian as against 45 British nurses do not have clients with neurosis (Tables 4.5 and 4.6).

This division between neurosis and psychosis does not take into account the variety of diagnoses that may be used in psychiatric services. In fact, it may be observed that there are 11 British nurses who do not have either group of client (of the 17 nurses with no neurotic patients only six had psychotic patients). Seemingly, these nurses target particular client groups such as the elderly – whose most frequent diagnosis is dementia praecox – or children. Moreover, it is certainly true that this broad division between neurosis and psychosis is more used in Italy, where this demarcation mainly indicates the border between 'hard' and 'soft' clients. Also, there is in Italy a widespread dislike of going in depth into diagnostic categories, in favour of qualitative reports about clients' needs and situation. It is thus that 'psychotic' and 'neurotic' become functional categories within the staff jargon indicating a broad division within services' clientele.

The majority of Italian clients are on nurses' caseloads indefinitely, whereas only 36.5% of British clients are on nurses' caseload for more than one year (Table 4.7).

Table 4.7 Number of clients spending various periods of time on nurses' caseloads (Mann–Whitney corrected for ties; two-tailed; $p = 0.000$; percentage in parentheses)

No.	UK (n = 63)	Italy (n = 56)
1–2 months	5 (7.9)	–
More than 2 months	14(22.2)	–
6 months	7(11.1)	12(21.4)
6 months–1 year	13(20.6)	–
More than 1 year	23(36.5)	–
Indefinitely	–	43(76.8)
No answer	1 (1.6)	1 (1.8)

This is a further significant difference that needs to be considered when comparing nurses' clientele in the two countries. It is again about clients' long-term care needs, which require a broad and long-lasting range of interventions.

The comparative analysis of nursing work practices confirms a trend towards specialization in British community psychiatric nursing that does not find an equivalent in Italy. British nurses' interventions relate to specific clinical areas, for which a knowledge base is usually necessary. On the other hand, Italian nurses make use of socially-oriented practices which do not generally require specialization and tend to produce a holistic style of intervention. The specific nursing clienteles involved are of course the reason for this difference. The majority of long-term clients served by Italian nurses have rehabilitation needs that require socially-oriented nursing models.

Table 4.8 indicates CPNs' practice in the two countries defined by 10 listed activities – speaking to clients, speaking to relatives, helping with the housework, taking part in leisure activities with clients, shopping with clients, monitoring medication, giving medication, counselling, family therapy and behaviour therapy.

It could be argued that the activity 'speaking to clients' tends to overlap with 'counselling'. Some British CPNs in fact said so, and thought their role was better described as 'counselling'. Hence the seven British nurses who appear not to 'speak to clients' chose to associate themselves with counselling activities. Such a distinction was considered to be useful with respect to the Italian sample. In Italy there is no specialization such as counselling, which is replaced by psychotherapy. However, some Italian nurses felt they were able to give counselling/psychotherapy, although not officially qualified to do so.

Table 4.8 Nurses' work practices: numbers of nurses engaging in particular activities with clients (percentage in parentheses)

Activity	UK (n = 63)	Italy (n = 56)	χ^2
Speaking to clients			
yes	56(89.0)	56(100)	
no	7(11.0)	0(0)	$p = 0.05$
Speaking to relatives			
yes	55(87.5)	52(93.0)	
no	8(12.5)	4(7.0)	–
Helping with housework			
yes	19(31.2)	33(59.0)	
no	44(68.8)	23(41.0)	$p = 0.01$
Taking part in leisure activities			
yes	27(45.3)	45(80.4)	
no	36(54.7)	11(19.6)	$p = 0.01$
Shopping with clients			
yes	26(42.0)	48(85.7)	
no	37(58.0)	8(14.3)	$p = 0.01$
Monitoring medication			
yes	55(87.5)	37(66.0)	
no	8(12.5)	19(34.0)	$p = 0.01$
Giving medication			
yes	36(57.8)	56(100)	
no	27(42.2)	0(0)	$p = 0.01$
Counselling			
yes	59(93.7)	23(41.0)	
no	4 (6.3)	33(59.0)	$p = 0.01$
Family therapy			
yes	35(56.2)	18(32.0)	
no	28(43.8)	38(68.0)	$p = 0.01$
Behaviour therapy			
yes	45(71.8)	17(30.4)	
no	18(28.2)	39(69.6)	$p = 0.01$

It is open to discussion whether 'speaking to clients' could in itself be 'therapeutic' and whether its practice could actually include counselling patterns of which nurses are not aware. Again it is important to comment upon the relationship between training and practice. On the one hand, lack of structured training in the Italian case tends to limit the number of specialized activities nurses carry out. On the other, loosely defined professional boundaries allow Italian nurses to undertake apparently deskilled activities like 'helping with housework', 'taking part in leisure activities with clients', 'shopping with clients' and 'giving medication'. Once again, it should not be taken for granted that the therapeutic outcome of these practices is not as valuable as that of family and behaviour therapy, i.e. could it not be that helping with the housework is a way of approaching family therapy? Table 4.8 indicates that there is a reverse trend in British and Italian answers from the least to the most specialized activities. The comparison proved to be significant for all the activities included apart from 'speaking to relatives'.

Nurses' performances among the Italian sample are mainly developed in the areas of speaking to clients, to relatives, taking part in leisure activities, going shopping, helping with housework and giving medication. Conversely, among the British sample there are high percentages of nurses who do not practise these interventions. Counselling, family therapy and behaviour therapy are among the activities practised least by Italian nurses and most by British nurses.

It is interesting to comment upon the difference between the activities 'monitoring' and 'giving medication'. All Italian nurses said they gave medication, whereas more than half of them said they did not monitor medication. In contrast, 85.7% of British nurses monitor medication and 27% do not give it. In order to understand this difference we must analyse how these two activities are perceived within the nursing professional culture in the two countries. It is necessary to understand that, for a long time, community psychiatric nurses both in Italy and in Britain have been associated with the administration of depot injections. This has been badly tolerated within the nursing professional culture in both countries, as it was felt to define the profession as merely executive rather than therapeutic. In fact, both British and Italian nurses ranked their activities by giving higher priorities to practices not directly associated with the administration of drugs. While giving medication is an executive task, the monitoring of medication requires specific skills usually ascribed to physicians. Although to the present writer's knowledge Italian nurses do monitor medication and actually change prescriptions before referring or consulting the doctor, they would rather not take direct responsibility for this. Conversely, British nurses seem to ascribe themselves to a higher professional position by increasing the monitoring task rather than the administration. This would confirm that the trend towards specialization identified in British nurses' practices is also reflected in their self-perceived professional identity. In contrast, the less specialized practices of Italian nurses still have some influence upon their perception as 'drug-supplying' professionals.

IDEOLOGIES OF CARE

Ideologies of nursing care have been investigated by asking CPNs from both samples to state their degree of agreement/disagreement with a number of statements representing five ideal ideologies of mental health/illness: the social, political, biological, psychological and critical ideologies. An example of CPNs' answers from each ideology of care will be reported here. However, it is important to note that overall results indicate that there is no prevalence of one ideological approach against another to distinguish British and Italian respondents. Rather, both British and Italian CPNs tend to consider mental illness as a multicausal phenomenon whose care requires a combination of social, psychological, biological and political approaches.

The comparison between the two sample groups indicates two major differences between nurses' attitudes towards mental illness.

1. Italian nurses tend to view community care as the only suitable option for the care of mental illness. The psychiatric hospital is in fact considered detrimental to mental health because of its stigmatizing character, its focus on illness rather than on health and the alienation of mentally distressed people caused by institutional life. On the other hand, British CPNs tend to view hospital and community care as alternative options for the treatment of mental illness. However, as far as their profession is concerned, they show preference towards the community setting, which allows them professional independence and creativity. This view may be partially due to the climate of professional uncertainty experienced by mental health workers in Britain, as a consequence of the move from the hospital to the community. Attitudes of resistance to change are in fact likely to emerge because of the substantial lack of professional involvement in government decisions about planning the move into the community. This reflects an important difference between the experience of British and Italian CPNs and certainly has some consequences on the philosophies of care promoted by the two professional groups.

2. The second main difference emerging from the findings can be identified in the nature of the responses provided by the two sample groups. While Italian CPNs tend to strongly support or oppose ideological statements, British respondents usually express moderate views both in the case of agreement and disagreement. These different attitudes are of a cultural nature. There is generally an element of 'drama' in the Italian culture which, mixed with idealism, generates radical views whenever political or social issues are at stake. This does not seem to be the case in Britain, where pragmatism is the prevailing attitude in social and political life. In part, this difference also explains the different character of the community care movements in the two countries.

Table 4.9 gives an example of CPNs' answers for each ideology of care. The analysis of nursing ideologies of care is in fact more complex, as CPNs answered about 70 ideological statements of which only five are illustrated here. Statement (1) represents the political ideology of mental health. It is self-explanatory, following the considerations expressed above. Statement (2)

Table 4.9 Number of nurses agreeing and disagreeing with various ideological statements about community psychiatric nursing (percentage in parentheses)

Position	UK (n = 59)	Italy (n = 50)
1. The psychiatric hospital does not have a curative function		
Strongly agree	4(6.8)	24(48.0)
Moderately agree	11(18.6)	12(24.0)
Slightly agree	7(11.9)	10(20.0)
Slightly disagree	6(10.2)	1(2.0)
Moderately disagree	16(27.1)	0(0)
Strongly disagree	14(23.7)	2(4.0)
No answer	1(1.7)	1(2.0)
2. Psychiatric nursing in the community has got the chance to become an eminent social and therapeutic role		
Strongly agree	31(52.5)	21(42.0)
Moderately agree	19(32.2)	20(40.0)
Slightly agree	4(6.8)	7(14.0)
Slightly disagree	3(5.1)	1(2.0)
No answer	2(3.4)	1(2.0)
3. Nurses are not competent to diagnose patients		
Strongly agree	2(3.4)	7(14.0)
Moderately agree	4(6.8)	11(22.0)
Slightly agree	4(6.8)	4(8.0)
Slightly disagree	2(3.4)	6(12.0)
Moderately disagree	25(42.4)	17(34.0)
Strongly disagree	21(35.6)	4(8.0)
No answer	1(1.7)	1(2.0)
4. Community care offers the best opportunity to develop therapeutic relationships with clients based on confidence and empathy		
Strongly agree	30(50.8)	25(50.0)
Moderately agree	23(39.0)	25(50.0)
Slightly agree	3(5.1)	0(0)
Slightly disagree	1(1.7)	0(0)
Moderately disagree	1(1.7)	0(0)
Strongly disagree	1(1.7)	0(0)
5. The shift to community care presents difficulties concerning the professional role and identity		
Strongly agree	10(16.9)	12(24.0)
Moderately agree	20(33.9)	15(30.0)
Slightly agree	16(27.1)	9(18.0)
Slightly disagree	1(1.7)	2(4.0)
Moderately disagree	6(10.2)	5(10.0)
Strongly disagree	5(8.5)	7(14.0)
No answer	1(1.7)	0(0)

represents the social ideology of mental health. It indicates a substantial agreement between the two samples about the opportunity that community work offers to the profession to undertake new, fulfilling developments. Statement (3) represents the biological ideology of mental health. It indicates an important difference between British and Italian CPNs concerning professional identity and role. Italian nurses are evidently less confident about their diagnostic capacities. Although this could be attributed to the different training of the two sample groups, it seems rather to point out the difficulty experienced by Italian nurses in perceiving themselves as independent practitioners. On the one hand, this may be due to the organization of work where they operate, which confers primary responsibility of care to the consultant psychiatrist. On the other hand, the lack of formal qualifications and standardized training certainly contributes to weakening the self-perceived professional identity.

Statement (4) represents the psychological approach to mental health. It again illustrates a convergency between the two samples, and confirms that community care is viewed as a positive professional experience by both British and Italian nurses. Statement (5) represents the critical approach to mental health. It shows a substantial agreement between the two groups on a topical issue in deinstitutionalization, i.e. the difficulty of undertaking major professional transformations during a stage of significant institutional change.

THE UNIQUENESS OF COMMUNITY PSYCHIATRIC NURSING

In the attempt to find elements common to the professional experience of British and Italian CPNs, respondents were also asked to describe those factors that confer to the job a unique character. The question was open-ended; the analysis of findings has therefore been qualitative. It emerges that the great majority of both British and Italian CPNs enjoy their job. There is something alive and enthusiastic in the description of the unique character of psychiatric nursing which can be considered as an indicator of the satisfaction towards the job. Also, there is a sort of pride in describing community psychiatric nursing in comparison with other nursing. There are two main groups of answers common to both samples which ascribe elements of uniqueness to the profession. Psychiatric nursing is an autonomous, brain-using, creative and self-directing job. It is client-centred rather than task oriented, like hospital nursing. The goals and organization of community work require the client, rather than the technical task, to be the specific care focus.

CPNs' descriptions depict a job that requires the individual to be able to decide on and operate non-codified intervention models. The non-clear-cut character of community psychiatric nursing is also a safeguard against routine; it is therefore challenging and intellectually stimulating. On the other hand, it can also be a source of stress and it certainly increases the difficulty of finding a specific professional identity. Among the perceived disadvantages of the profession, in fact, British nurses indicate the non-clear-cut character of the job and Italian nurses the high levels of stress experienced in everyday practice.

CONCLUSIONS

The analysis of findings indicates the existence of two different models of community psychiatric nursing in Britain and Italy, which are to be linked with the cultural and historical approaches characterizing community care in the two countries. In Britain the prevailing model is of progressive specialization. The development of new approaches to the care of mental illness is taking place through the differentiation of professional competences, of which community psychiatric nursing is perhaps the most obvious example. The acknowledgement of the increasing complexity of the needs of mentally distressed people in the community has brought about a prompt definition and division of professional roles, competences, target groups and aims of services. This is shown by the number of specialized functions which the British CPNs in this study perform, as well as by their educational advancement and organizational style. On the other hand, the Italian care model aims at being comprehensive, so that services tend to be inclusive rather than exclusive. Mental health care is not differentiated by client group, nor by professional group. While interprofessional hierarchy is quite limited – not only within nursing – there is a prevalence of an organizational hierarchy whereby CMHCs hold the institutional mandate to plan the care packages and define the competences of the other community agencies. The community network is generally based on the CMHC which is the fulcrum of the system. Other agencies, like day centres and residential homes, depend upon the CMHC and in general the same professional team rotates between the different structures. In order to maintain the complexity and holistic character of this care model, Italian CPNs need to avoid differentiation. Findings show that CPNs competences are of a holistic nature, with a substantial lack of standardization.

Yet there are interesting similarities between the experiences of British and Italian community psychiatric nurses. Respondents from both samples agree that their community role is significantly different from the past hospital role. Community psychiatric nursing is a client-centred profession that allows professional independence and creativity. In terms of professional development, the shift from task-oriented to client-centred activities implies the acquisition of new care approaches whose focus is more on social and psychological interventions than executive practices. This is particularly significant to the professionalization of psychiatric nursing. It means that CPNs have succeeded in gaining one of the new care market areas which developed as a consequence of deinstitutionalization. It is nevertheless fundamental that these new developments in the practice of community psychiatric nursing are adequately acknowledged through institutionalized training programmes for CPNs. Both British and Italian CPNs need to concentrate their professional efforts on obtaining educational advancements which can appropriately support and back up their practice. This is an important stage in establishing a new psychiatric nursing professionalism. The 36-week post-qualifying community psychiatric nursing course in Britain must be mandatory to achieve this. In Italy, nurses need to actively promote the establishment of specific and institutionalized CPN courses. These are steps necessary to represent the profession within the psychiatric care professional market and to increase the mechanisms of identification within the profession. There are, in fact, difficulties at the level of professional identity for both groups. The non-clear-cut character of community work is perceived as both an advantage and a disadvantage. On the one hand, it enhances nurses' autonomy; on the other hand, the unclear definition of professional tasks produces uncertainty at the levels of professional identity and roles. While this perception is common to both British and Italian nurses, the conditions that support it are different. The difficulties endured by British CPNs are possibly due to the transition from a hospital task-centred role to a loosely defined, although more rewarding, community practice. The fact that British respondents maintain the positive function of psychiatric hospitals, although regarding community care as a privileged professional opportunity, may be significant. Specialization is another means to control uncertainty: it defines a specific client group and the related areas of professional intervention. Yet specialization is not obviously enough, since British CPNs still complain about the non-clear-cut character of the job.

Italian CPNs lack a means of identification with the profession at the structural level, as there are no specific courses for psychiatric nursing in hospital nor in the community. On the operational side, community-established nursing practice does not meet with an adequate educational support and professional status.

An answer to the questions laid out in the introductory section (what does professionalization mean: does it necessarily mean specialization? and what is the role of CPN in the transition from the hospital to the community?) must take into account both the differences detected crossnationally between British and Italian CPNs and the similarities. While the differences stem from historical and cultural developments in community care in the two countries, the similarities possibly outline universal characteristics in the role of nursing at a stage of significant institutional transformation.

That community psychiatric nursing is moving towards the establishment of a new professionalism seems to be confirmed by the findings from both samples. The implementation of community-based psychiatric nursing has consistently changed the traditional hospital role ascribed to the occupation. Specialization appears at this stage a necessary condition for the institutional acknowledgement of this new professionalism. Nevertheless, both British and Italian CPNs need to avoid overlapping with other community professions, like social work and psychology, whose interventions are also becoming increasingly important in community care.

Counselling, psychotherapy, behaviour and family therapy are among the main areas of specialization undertaken by British CPNs. While it is certainly useful to develop professional skills in these fields, it may be important not to concentrate all the professional effort exclusively in such areas. This would not, in fact, promote the identification of a specific and unique contribution of community psychiatric nursing to the speciality of psychiatry. At the other end of the continuum there are Italian CPNs whose only specialism is dealing with the holistic character of community care. These two different care models have as common features that they focus on client-centred rather than task-centred activities, and enjoy a considerable degree of professional autonomy and independence. A pathway to professionalism for both groups might therefore be to increase the client-centred nature of the job by focusing on a new and important clientele in community care – continued care clients.

To a large extent the success or failure of community care depends on the ability of professionals to provide adequate services to continued care clients. The challenge is to develop care approaches able to meet needs that can no longer be easily boxed within clinical categories, and instead require a holistic range of interventions. The development of community care has contributed to rendering these needs more visible, and at the same time has highlighted the inadequacy of hospital-based care models in providing a homogeneous response to such needs. Community psychiatric nursing seems to be the most obvious link between the traditional hospital psychiatry and the future of community care. The level of specialization of psychiatric occupations like social work, psychology and psychiatry is such that their contributions to the care of continued care clients can only be partial. Otherwise, they would lose their specialist character. The only occupation which, at this stage, can afford to embrace a holistic approach is community psychiatric nursing – because its new professional traits are not yet defined and because it can accompany the transition from the hospital to the community.

This hypothesis is in itself a paradox. It says that the specialization of CPN has to be oriented towards holistic practices. The obvious risk is to produce a professional condition similar to that of Italian CPNs, who have a holistic approach but a low professional status. This occurs as a consequence of community psychiatric nursing's subordinate position within psychiatry, as the power of status and decisions is still held by psychiatrists. A necessary step is then to acknowledge that the contribution of CPN is complementary and not subordinated to that of other occupations within the field. The professional and institutional role of community psychiatric nursing is therefore to make it acceptable and obvious that psychiatry is no longer just the science of psychiatrists. The rehabilitation of continued care clients requires the needs of people to be tackled through a normalization approach. In order to undertake this task properly, psychiatry also has to be normalized. It is perhaps for CPNs to promote this new psychiatric ideology. In order not to render the normalization approach detrimental to the profession it is important that the provision of holistic practices becomes standardized. It has to be a method, a model, and not the result of improvisation or a lack of professional competence. Italian nurses may acquire from their British colleagues the ability to transform everyday practices into procedures that can be monitored and evaluated. This is the strength of the British approach and is a fundamental requirement for services directed towards people, whose well-being needs to be the ultimate aim of professional practice. British CPNs, on the other hand, may need to improve their confidence in community practice by acknowledging the relevant potential of communtiy care, as compared to the hospital, as well as acknowledging that psychiatric care is undergoing a major epistemological transformation of which they are the vanguard.

REFERENCE

Strauss, A. (1964) *Psychiatric Ideologies and Institutions*, The Free Press of Glencoe, Glencoe, IL.

FURTHER READING

British and Italian community psychiatric nursing

Battaglia, G. (1987) The expanding role of the nurse and the contracting role of the hospital in Italy. *International Journal of Social Psychiatry*, **33**, 115–18.
Brooker, C. (1985) Community Mental Health Services in Italy. The implications for community psychiatric nurses in the UK. *Community Psychiatric Nursing Journal*, **May/June**.
Pollock, L. (1989) *Community Psychiatry Nursing. Myth or Reality?* Royal College of Nursing, London.
Savio, M. (1991) Psychiatric nursing in Italy: an extinguished profession or an emerging professionalism? *International Journal of Social Psychiatry*, **37**, 293–9.
White, E. (1990) *Community Psychiatric Nursing. The 1990 CPN Survey*, CPNA Publications, London.
White, E. (1991) The historical development of the educational preparation of CPNs, in *Community Psychiatric Nursing. A Research Perspective*, (ed. C. Brooker), Chapman & Hall, London.
Zani, B. (1984) *Da custodi dei matti ad operatori di salute mentale*, Franco Angeli, Milano.

Professionalization

Jackson, J. (1970) *Professions and Professionalisation*, Cambridge University Press, Cambridge.

Ramon, S. (1986) The making of a professional culture: professionals in psychiatry in Britain and Italy since 1945. Cross-National Comparative Research Seminar, University of Aston, Birmingham.

Ideology

Thompson, T. (1984) *Studies in the Theory of Ideology*, Polity Press, Cambridge.

Organization

Scott, R.W. and Black, L.B. (1986) *The Organization of Mental Health Services. Societal and Community System*, Sage Publications, London.

CHAPTER FIVE

Telephone work with CPN service users

Kate Wilson, Anthony Butterworth and

Anne Williams

INTRODUCTION

This chapter is based on Department of Health funded research, conducted between November 1989 and May 1993 at the School of Nursing Studies, University of Manchester. The project explored the telephone work of three groups of community nurses: community psychiatric nurses (CPNs), district nurses (DNs) and health visitors (HVs). This chapter focuses on the work of CPNs but data relating to DNs and HVs will be introduced where relevant.

A major stimulus for this project was the proliferation of voluntary sector telephone helplines over recent years, many of which deal with mental health and psychosocial concerns (Bryan, 1988). It also followed, and complemented, Department of Health funded research into telephone consultation in general practice (Hallam, 1989). As it was the first large-scale British investigation into the role of the telephone in community nursing, the scope of the research was appropriately broad. The following areas of discussion are included in this chapter: call volumes, time spent on telephone work, who calls and why, nurse-initiated calls, facilities and possible developments. Discussion is preceded by a brief overview of key literature and an account of study research methods.

The project focused on the work of registered nurses only. There was also an intention to restrict study to generic nurses in all three groups. However, as the definition of specialization in CPN practice was found to be problematic (White, 1990a), it proved necessary to use an operational definition of the term 'specialist'. This definition and its associated rationale will be presented later in this chapter.

A REVIEW OF THE LITERATURE

A literature review was carried out during late 1989 and early 1990. At this time, apart from passing references in books which describe overall practice (Parnell, 1978; Dunnell and Dobbs, 1982), no published literature on CPN telephone work could be found. Of the three groups of nurses studied, it seemed that only health visiting had produced publications specific to telephone work with service users. These describe helpline-mediated out-of-hours schemes (Greenwood, 1979; Beech, 1981; Rawdon Smith, 1984; Angel, Nicholl and Amatiello, 1988) rather than everyday telephone practice.

The paucity of British nursing literature led to a search for relevant publications from international and multidisciplinary sources. A large volume of literature was identified, some of it describing the telephone work of hospital, clinic and visiting nurses (Cave, 1989; Munroe and Natale, 1982; Hampson, 1989). This included only one reference to psychiatric nursing in the community: O'Donnell and George (1977) mention that two community mental health nurses formed part of the professional/lay team staffing a crisis intervention line in Illinois. Much of the literature describes crisis and counselling helplines, some run by 'multidisciplinary health professionals' (Winogrond and Mirrasou, 1983), but many others by the voluntary or 'not for profit' sector (Varah, 1973; Tapp, Slaikeu and Tulkin, 1974; Knowles, 1979; Drummond, 1980; Hornblow and Sloane, 1980; Hirsch, 1981; Davies, 1982; Elkins and Cohen, 1982; Walfish, 1983).

Many of these authors argue that the telephone facilitates access to health care. O'Donnell and George (1977) describe it as a 'gate' to services and an 'essential preliminary screening device'. However, access may not be equal for all. Winogrond and Mirassou (1983) state that only 9% of clients aged 70 and over self-referred (as opposed to 55% of those aged 40 and under) and attribute this to a high frequency of disabling psychological problems amongst older clients. Nevertheless, such clients quite frequently gained help through family members contacting the helpline. Several articles, addressing both physical and psychosocial health issues, suggest that 'telephoners' are characteristically white, middle-class, middle-aged females (Pope, Yoshioka and Greenlick, 1971; Rainey, 1985; Slevin *et al.*, 1988). Two studies may be of relevance here: Diseker, Michielutte and Morrison (1980) show that, while economically disadvantaged people may often be unaware of services, the call-rate of those who are aware may be comparable to that of the middle-classes; Wilkinson, Mirand and Graham (1976), in a simple experiment, demonstrate a dramatic rise in call-rates in a town saturated with publicity as compared to a control town.

Much of the literature describing voluntary helplines discusses the need for training in telephone communication skills (Tapp, Slaikeu and Tulkin, 1974: Knowles, 1979; Drummond, 1980; Davies, 1982; Elkins and Cohen, 1982; Walfish, 1983). Most of these authors favour thorough initial preparation followed by supervised practice and inservice training. Goodman and Perrin (1978), Curtis and Talbot (1981), Evens and Curtis (1983) and McDonald (1987) discuss similar issues with regard to health professionals. McDonald suggests that nurses who learn telephone communication skills through experience alone may give poor service to early callers.

Most of the publications identified during the initial literature search describe helplines dealing with psychosocial concerns. During the course of the project, articles were published that discuss telephone support services for carers of people with dementia (Coyne, 1991; O'Donovan, 1993). O'Donovan's article, although written from a British psychiatric nursing perspective, describes a helpline set up by an elderly mentally ill service rather than a CPN service.

METHODS

A national postal survey of CPNs

CPN contacts for each district health authority (DHA), listed in an existing publication (White, 1990b), were approached and asked to provide details of all CPN fieldworkers. In this way, 188 (98%) English DHAs could be contacted; 178 (95%) of the DHAs contacted replied and furnished details (93% of all English DHAs). Lists of CPNs were scrutinized and all but registered nurses were excluded. CPNs working in forensic, child psychiatry and drug and alcohol services were defined as specialists and excluded, as these specialisms were thought to have adopted practice styles distinct from those of generic practitioners. Eligible CPNs were numbered and a simple random sample was selected by computer generation of 500 random numbers. Since the population of English CPNs (generic and specialist) could be estimated at approximately 4291 (White, 1990a), this represented a more than adequate sample.

A questionnaire, which had been developed and piloted with the aid of local CPNs, was dispatched to each nurse in the sample, along with a covering letter and a reply-paid envelope. Non-respondents were sent a second questionnire, letter and envelope 1 month later. Following this, the number of returned questionnaires totalled 380, a 76% response rate.

The findings on several key characteristics of respondents (including gender ratio, ratio of part-timers to full-timers and base locations) showed close agreement with those of White (1990a) and lend support for the representativeness of CPN respondents. For example, 55% of respondents were female, which compares with 54.2% of White's respondents. The national survey was also conducted among 504 DNs and 676 HVs but, unfortunately, sampling procedures were problematic, making it more difficult to claim representativeness for the respondents and data. Response rates for DNs and HVs were 77% and 81% respectively.

An interview survey of CPNs

A purposive sample of five CPN respondents to the postal survey who appeared to have a positive attitude to telephone consultation was selected (along with five similar DNs and HVs). Survey data suggested that 'telephone-positive' nurses were able to discuss both the advantages and disadvantages of telephone use, whereas those at the 'telephone negative' end of the spectrum tended to place more emphasis on disadvantages alone. It was also thought that telephone-positive nurses might provide some interesting models of good practice. These taped focused interviews were conducted at nurses' bases.

Call-logging

Interviewees were asked to log all telephone calls to and from service users over a period of seven consecutive working days. Numerical data wTere generated but, in view of the non-random nature of the sample, this was used to provide further insights into the work of the interview sample and was not intended to be generalizable to the larger population of generic CPNs.

A survey of service users

Permission to interview the five CPNs (plus the five DNs and five HVs) and to survey their clients was sought from service managers, who also provided contacts for local ethics committees. Negotiations with ethics committees proved to be lengthy: in the case of one CPN they had to be abandoned. After discussing sampling strategies with nurses, it was decided that they should distribute questionnaires to consecutive clients seen both at home and in clinics for the period of a month (a convenience sample). This method had the possible disadvantage of introducing bias through nurses 'selecting out' certain clients. In addition, a few clients seen less frequently than monthly may have been missed by this sampling strategy.

Questionnaires were short (17 items) and concentrated on the accessibility of nurses by telephone. Respondents were invited to make general comments on telephoning nurses in a final open-ended question. Where clients were unable to complete questionnaires themselves, responses from carers or significant others were accepted. Completed questionnaires were posted direct to the School of Nursing Studies in prepaid envelopes.

Response rates varied from nurse to nurse: the four CPNs had rates of 37%, 58%, 85% and 94%. In cases where there was less than a 50% response rate questionnaires were not subjected to numerical analysis. Client survey data were used to further illuminate the work of the nurses interviewed.

FINDINGS

The project yielded a large amount of quantitative and qualitative data. This chapter attempts to balance presentation of a selection of largely quantitative findings on current telephone practice and facilities with discussion of qualitative data about possible future developments in telephone work.

Volume of telephone calls

Respondents to the postal survey estimated the number of telephone calls received from and made to service users per week: the data obtained are presented in Figure 5.1. A total of 31% of CPNs estimated that they received five or fewer calls from service users per week. At the other end of the scale, only 5% received in excess of 20 calls. While 21% of CPNs estimated that they made five or fewer calls to service users per week, 9% made more than

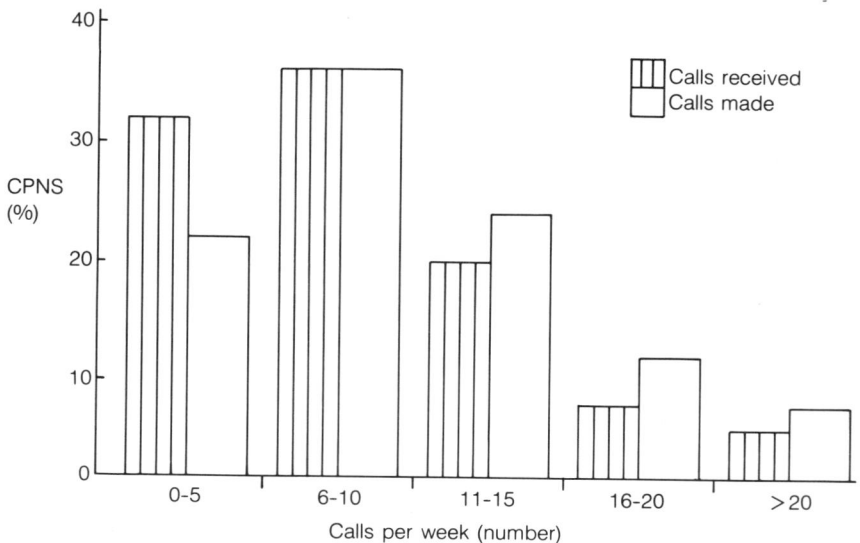

Figure 5.1 Postal survey: number of calls received from and made to service users per week by percentage of CPNs.

20. This, along with the rest of the data in Figure 5.1, suggests that CPNs initiate rather more calls to service users than they receive. Among DNs and HVs, numbers of incoming and outgoing calls seem to be more balanced. HVs seem to make and receive the highest number of calls and DNs the lowest, with CPNs occupying an intermediate position.

Time spent on telephone work

CPNs also estimated the length of time that they spent per week on handling calls from and making calls to service users. The median time spent handling incoming calls was 1.5 hours per week (range 0–9 hours). The median time spent on making calls to service users was 2.0 hours (range 0–10 hours). This higher median time for CPN-initiated calls than calls from users is congruent with call volume data. Parnell (1978) reported that CPNs spent an average of 1 hour 56 minutes per week in professional discussion by telephone (all incoming/outgoing and service user/interprofessional calls).

The median value for the proportion of total working time spent on telephone calls, both to and from service users, was 8.8% (range 0–62.5%). CPNs were reported to be spending 5% of their working time on telephone calls in 1980 (Dunnell and Dobbs, 1982). This seems consistent with the findings of Parnell quoted above. Postal survey data are congruent with the findings of both authors, showing similar increases in time spent (81% increase) and percentage of working time spent (76% increase) on telephone calls since the late 1970s/early 1980s. These increases appear to be substantial, especially in view of the fact that the earlier figures refer to all calls, whereas the postal survey figures refer only to telephone calls to and from service users.

Who calls and why?

The CPNs interviewed said that they received more calls from carers and significant others than clients themselves. Call logging tended to support this: 57% of calls made to CPNs were from people described as carers, relatives or friends. Interviews and call-logging identified that these calls were frequently concerned with the deterioration of clients with chronic mental illness or dementia. Those calling on their own behalf tended to be 'the worried well' and 'neurotic people who are more able to speak for themselves'. Only 3% of the calls logged by CPNs were from people who were not known clients or their carers, relatives and friends.

CPN interviewees identified four groups of people as being less likely (or unlikely) to possess private telephones: the elderly, people on low incomes, people in sheltered housing and homeless people in hotels or hostels. It was also suggested that such clients were reluctant to use payphones when trying to contact CPNs. However, data from the postal survey demonstrated no correlation between CPNs' estimates of levels of telephone ownership in their caseloads and the estimated number of calls received per week.

Nurse-initiated calls

Interview data show that many nurse-initiated calls were made in response to messages left by users or requests for help made during previous calls and visits. These calls were closely related to the types of user-initiated call discussed above. Calls made to monitor the progress of people and situations also featured quite strongly. Most of the remaining calls were made for organizational purposes, to follow up missed appointments or to provide support.

CPN survey respondents estimated the percentage of nurse-initiated calls which were made for organizational purposes only. A median value of 65% was obtained (range 0–100%). This was a somewhat higher percentage than for either DNs (50%) or HVs (55%). The CPNs interviewed were largely in favour of visiting by appointment, some feeling that it improved time management by reducing no reply visits. Making appointments by telephone was generally held to be speedier and more effective than making them in writing.

The nurses interviewed had diverse views about following up no reply visits and non-attenders. One CPN spoke at length on the subject: she felt that following up injection clinic non-attenders by telephone, rather than in person, made for 'a less threatening service'. This was related to her commitment to supportive, rather than coercive, CPN practice.

Interviewees suggested that supportive work was often carried out during calls that were ostensibly organizational or served some other instrumental purpose. One CPN, however, regularly made supportive calls to discharged clients. Of CPN respondents to the postal survey, 11(3%) said that they took part in telephone monitoring or support schemes: these were frequently aimed at monitoring discharged clients/people in remission or supporting carers. Whether these schemes were run by individuals or larger numbers of nurses cannot be determined.

Office and telephone facilities

In response to the postal survey 336 (88%) CPNs said that they worked in a shared office. CPNs shared with a median of three others (range 0–19). In this respect they were quite similar to HVs, but both groups were better served than DNs who shared with a median of six others (range 0–37). When nurses were asked about difficulties in carrying out telephone consultation at their bases, noise emerged as the most frequent difficulty for all three nurse groups (mentioned by 61% of CPNs, 73% of DNs and 56% of HVs). Lack of privacy and confidentiality was mentioned by 42% of CPNs; this was the second most frequent difficulty for CPNs and HVs. One of the CPNs interviewed, who shared with seven others, highlighted the problem of office-sharing:

> It is a large room ... it is extremely noisy and you are really trying to listen to somebody on the other end. The line may be bad or they may be talking quietly or they may be distressed or something. You have got the phone jammed up against one ear, your finger stuck in the other ear and eventually you go and yell at somebody 'Oh, stop fiddling with the filing cabinet; I am trying to listen here!'

A total of 45% of CPN respondents to the postal survey said that they would like a 'quiet room' for telephone work. One CPN interviewed had access to a 'side room' which she was able to use when making long or particularly confidential calls. Sometimes, difficult incoming calls were transferred to this room. Another CPN stated that a reduction in the number of people sharing her office, and a consequent increase in privacy, had helped to lessen her sense of inhibition when dealing with client problems over the telephone.

Postal survey data relating to CPNs' accessibility by telephone are presented in Table 5.1.

Comparable HV and DN data suggest that CPNs have rather better telephone facilities than their colleagues. In particular, only 28% of DN and 22% of HV respondents had the use of an answering machine. More CPNs worked in rooms with direct lines, more had message-taking systems (both in

Table 5.1 Accessibility of CPNs by telephone (percentage in parentheses)

CPNs based in office with phone	379(100)
CPNs based in office with direct line	284(75)
Use of answering machine	231(61)
Presence of message-taking system	
during normal working hours*	353(93)
out of hours*	254(67)
Use of mobile device	100(26)
pager	92(24)
car/mobile phone	2(1)
Existence of telephone contact times	187(49)
CPN service contactable out of hours	
always	23(6)
sometimes	66(17)
Home number given to selected clients or carers	25(7)

*including answering machine

and out of normal working hours) and fewer cited problems with message-takers' skills. Although fewer CPNs than DNs (42%) had mobile devices, the comparable figure for HVs was only 1%.

However, CPNs lagged behind their colleagues when it came to contact provision for users. For instance, 68% of DN respondents and 80% of HV respondents had telephone contact times. The proportion of CPN services not contactable out of normal working hours (76%) was slightly higher than for HV services (73%) and much higher than for DN services (33%). A much lower percentage of CPNs gave their home telephone number to selected clients and carers than DNs (62%) or HVs (64%). While there may be good reasons for such differences (particularly in the case of giving home numbers), the net result may be inferior access. However the existence of better telephone facilities, such as adequate human and electronic message-taking, may render other arrangements for contact less important, especially during normal working hours.

When CPNs' perceptions of their accessibility to service users were cross-tabulated with their type of base (health centre, GP surgery, health clinic, hospital, mental health resource centre or other) no relationship was found. Of the CPN respondents to the postal survey, 269 (71%) judged their accessibility by telephone to be satisfactory. The remaining respondents perceived few access problems. The major ones are listed in Table 5.2.

Table 5.2 Major access problems (based on responses from 100 CPNs; percentage in parentheses)

Nurse out most of the day	55(50)
No/poor out-of-hours cover	18(16)
Telephone lines engaged	16(15)
No/poor message-taking	14(13)

The two most frequently cited access problems relate to contact provision rather than telephone facilities. However, in answer to questions about improvements in telephone facilities, sizeable minorities of CPN respondents thought the improvements detailed in Table 5.3 desirable.

In their desire for increased handsets, direct lines and car/mobile phones, CPNs may be more concerned with their ability to make outgoing calls than with their accessibility to service users. This seems probable, given that the majority of CPN respondents felt that their accessibility was satisfactory and that CPNs seem to make more calls to service users than they receive.

Table 5.3 Desirable improvements desired to CPN telephone access (percentage in parentheses)

More telephone handsets in office	154(41)
Direct lines/more direct lines	155(41)
Answering machine	63(16)
Improvement in message-taking cover	102(27)
Mobile device	189(50)
car/mobile phone	109(29)
Change of mobile device	50(16)
to car/mobile phone	33(9)

DEVELOPMENTS IN TELEPHONE WORK

Only 30% of CPN respondents to the postal survey answered in the affirmative when asked if they wished to develop their use of telephone work (the figures for DNs and HVs were 29% and 45% respectively). However, some nurses who answered in the negative went on to comment that they would like telephone training or favoured the setting up of telephone duty systems. Spontaneous comments, exemplified by the following, suggested a possible reason for this: 'I do not think phone contact can ever replace face-to-face contact, although it has its uses.' Concern about the motives of the research project is implicit in comments made by members of all three nurse groups and may have affected responses to questions such as that on development of telephone work.

Special telephone services

Not surprisingly, the majority of the nurses interviewed expressed a desire to make themselves and/or their particular nursing service more accessible to service users by telephone through improving or extending nurses' availability as well as improving facilities.

In some cases nurses were keen to give greater telephone access to the community in general. Many of them discussed the setting up of duty systems and advice lines, where a nurse would be available by telephone either throughout each working day or for specific publicized sessions in the week. Some interviewees also spoke about out-of-hours telephone support and advice services.

In response to the postal survey of nurses 21 (6%) CPN respondents, six (2%) DN respondents and 42 (8%) HV respondents said that they were involved in helpline-type telephone schemes. The majority of CPN schemes were aimed at all known clients and carers (and sometimes members of the public) rather than targeted on particular client groups. Most of the CPNs interviewed were reluctant to identify specific groups of clients who might benefit from telephone schemes. The following comment about resources was also fairly typical:

> I think voluntary organizations like Making Space and Mind are setting up telephone helplines and I think that is excellent. There are helplines for depressives. I don't really think that running helplines for specific illnesses is an effective use of our resources.

Another CPN had a close relationship with a local Alzheimer's Society group who were in the process of setting up a helpline. Although she was prepared to collect information, compile lists of contacts and get involved in training issues, she said that actual participation in the helpline was 'impractical' because of the size of her caseload.

One CPN, based in a community mental health centre, participated in a multidisciplinary duty system which served both telephone callers and people dropping in during normal working hours. This system was suffering because of staff shortages and was inoperative on the day that the interviewer visited. The CPN had a clear picture of her ideal telephone service: it would be run exclusively by CPNs from 10 a.m. to 10 p.m. seven days per week. For security reasons, it would be based at the local hospital, served by a direct line rather than the switchboard. An answering machine would be in operation between 10 p.m. and 10 a.m. to give information, including the time the service reopened and alternative sources of help. She estimated that this might require an extra two whole-time equivalent CPNs, who might be employed as joint appointees between the regular CPN service and the telephone scheme. This would allow them to keep their skills updated while safeguarding time for their specialist role. The CPN felt that this service was unlikely to materialize in the prevailing 'economic climate'. However, she said:

> There are plans within Redville to look at a 24-hour system for help, because quite often it is 8 or 9 o'clock at night when people call for help. ... I think it would be a good idea if the CPNs were involved. It is very much problem-solving at the front line.

A carer of one of this CPN's clients wrote enthusiastically about this projected scheme, in response to the client survey:

> A number that husbands, wives, relatives who have anyone suffering psychiatric problems, relapses etc. could contact 24 hours a day is a **damn good idea**.

This respondent's wife had recently relapsed during the night. The locum doctor who dealt with the relapse was 'not much help'. The respondent had since attended a meeting about the setting up of a 24-hour telephone service in Redville. Another of the Redville nurse's clients commented: 'Everyone should be given a telephone number to ring, if they are ill, day or night.' Only service users from Redville made comments about special telephone services. This may suggest that users do not consider that such provision is possible unless personal experience leads them to think otherwise. Whether limited resources would allow this scheme to work better than the current multidisciplinary duty system remains to be seen.

Although duty systems and advice lines may be an attractive concept, the current workloads of many community nurses may make participation difficult or impossible. Other structural factors, such as poor telephone facilities, may also cause difficulties. Duty systems may only be possible at large bases with adequate staff numbers. Cooperation between nurses from different bases (or even from different services) was not discussed by the CPNs interviewed, but may be feasible if participating nurses refer some callers' queries and problems on to the most appropriate nurse or service. However, the organization of such schemes may prove problematical, particularly since the advent of GP purchasing. Neither the existing literature nor this piece of research has produced clear evidence that duty systems and similar schemes are cost-effective. In view of this, liaison with voluntary helplines, including those dealing with specific disorders, may prove a useful alternative: this subject will be discussed further.

Publicity

Many of the nurses interviewed recognized the need to advertise telephone schemes and/or encourage clients to call, if such schemes were to prove worthwhile. Some also spoke about the need to publicize their general availability by telephone. The question of appropriate publicity is dependent on numerous factors, including nurses' modes of attachment and, in the case of CPNs (and DNs), policies relating to 'self' or 'open' referral, issues which proved too complex to explore fully. It seems that most nurses can do a 'one-off' consultation with members of the public from the appropriate practice, geographical area or sector but must get 'medical back-up' before further intervention. Nurses who are governed by local policies stating that they cannot accept open referrals are unlikely, however, to publicize their telephone numbers and calling arrangements to anyone but their existing clients. In response to the postal survey, 276 (73%) CPN respondents stated that they accepted self-referrals. The postal survey also found that 49% of the CPN respondents who accepted self-referrals did not publicize this fact.

Three of the CPNs interviewed accepted self-referrals and yielded copious data on the subject of publicity. They discussed the subjects of attracting appropriate callers and concerns about misuse. The CPN who wanted to run a duty line was, nonetheless, concerned that publicity about the CPN service might cause it to be 'swamped'.

> The people we aim to target, on the whole, are the chronic mentally ill – nobody wants to know about those. People with neurosis are well able to say 'There is something wrong with me' and my feeling is that, if we advertise, we will get a lot more because the sort of things that will probably go out in the adverts are 'Feeling under the weather? Under stress? Can't cope?' Well, that is all of us, isn't it?

She went on to consider whether just the helpline could be publicized, as distinct from the CPN service as a whole:

> I think you could publicize the helpline. . . . I think you could blitz the whole of Redville with 'Telephone Helpline Run by Community Nurse'. It is difficult really, because if you put the word 'psychiatric' in, you'll put a lot of people off. If you don't put 'psychiatric' in, you are going to get [calls saying] 'My mother's got leg ulcers'. . . . I think that could clog the system up and it might put people off using it.

She eventually decided that the best plan might be to give leaflets to professionals, such as doctors and psychologists, who could hand them out to appropriate patients and clients. A helpline publicized in this way is, however, unlikely to be used by the public as a first means of contact with health services.

The other two CPNs who had open referral policies made similar comments about publicizing their services, and in particular their availability by phone:

> Well, it is an open referral system . . . but we don't advertise this. We just haven't got the facilities . . . we would be inundated. It is sad really that we haven't got the capacity to do what we know we want to do . . .
>
> If we did shout about it [the service] a lot we might very well get a lot more referrals – more than we could possibly cope with. I mean, we are running about as hard as we can at the moment.

The first of these CPNs was consultant-attached and said that there was sometimes tension between this fact and the open referral policy. The second CPN was geographically attached but said that the vast majority of his referrals came from 'the triumvirate: Consultant, GP, Social Services'. It is perhaps surprising to note, given the above interview data, that 31 (12%) CPN respondents to the postal survey who accepted self-referrals advertised themselves in public places (such as shops and libraries). This is a higher proportion than either DNs (3%) or HVs (11%). Perhaps even more surprisingly, 88 (33%) of these CPNs also advertised in practice leaflets, as opposed to 73 (22%) of the equivalent DNs. In addition, 28 (10%) of CPNs made use of practice posters, as opposed to 23 (7%) of the DNs.

One consultant-attached CPN who did not officially accept self-referrals was, however, able to give one-off advice before seeking medical back-up.

She was very concerned about 'late referrals', where people with Alzheimer's disease and their carers were not referred to the service until a crisis occurred. She thought, in this context, that publicizing CPN availability by phone 'would probably be ideal but probably totally impractical . . . there just aren't the resources, although maybe there should be'.

It was this CPN who spoke about her involvement in a helpline to be set up by the Alzheimer's Society. She hoped that this would be well-publicized and would screen callers, referring appropriate cases to the CPN service. This scheme echoes the lay/professional venture described by O'Donnell and George (1977). Community nurses who wish to encourage self-referral by telephone (but who realize that they do not have the resources to publicize themselves directly, staff a helpline or deal with large volumes of calls) might take note of this collaboration with the voluntary sector.

Some of the nurses interviewed suggested that most callers were people who knew and trusted them, and that such people chose to telephone them specifically because of this. Postal survey data were used to investigate this idea further. Nurses' length of service in their present post was cross-tabulated wih their estimates of numbers of calls from service users. Results show that longer-established CPNs and HVs had significantly greater number of calls from users ($p = 0.03$ by chi-square test). In the case of DNs, however, this correlation did not exist. This may be related, at least in part, to callers who phone about psychosocial concerns, where issues of familiarity and trust may be particularly important. Interview data suggest that many of those calling DNs with such concerns are carers of terminally ill people, who are likely to be on DNs' caseloads for a limited time. The above findings seem to lend some support to the idea that familiarity breeds calls, although it must be recognized that volumes of incoming calls are based on nurses' estimates. If it is true that people phone community nurses mainly because they know them, publicity measures may be of little value in encouraging unknown sections of the population to use nurses as first sources of advice. However, it is equally possible that appropriate publicity could increase awareness of community nurses (and alter people's concepts of them), thus changing predominant patterns of contact and self-referral. Carefully monitored experiments with publicity might show which of these is true.

Telephone communication skills and training

Although the majority of respondents to the postal survey of community nurses said that they had received communication skills training, few had been given training in telephone-specific skills. CPNs were rather better served in this respect than their colleagues. Figures relating to these two variables are given in Table 5.4.

Table 5.4 Postal survey results: numbers of CPNs, DNs and HVs who have had communication skills training and telephone skills training (m/c = missing cases; percentage in parentheses)

Training	Nurse group		
	CPNs (n = 380)	DNs (n = 388)	HVs n = 545)
Communication skills	322(86)	294(77)	459(85)
	5 m/c	4 m/c	5 m/c
Telephone skills	52(14)	18(5)	42(8)
	6 m/c	4 m/c	4 m/c

Most commonly, CPNs had received communication skills input during RMN training; for DNs and HVs the predominant setting was community nurse training. The survey questionnaire did not specifically seek information on the circumstances under which telephone training had been received; however, a few CPNs made unsolicited comments such as 'as a Samaritan volunteer', 'I am a trained secretary' and 'not as a health authority employee'. None of the respondents commented that they had received telephone training in nursing settings. Several respondents to the postal survey, including CPNs, made comments similar to the following: 'I feel I need further training and supervision with telephone counselling work'. No comments were made implying that telephone training was unnecessary or irrelevant.

As might be expected, the telephone-positive nurses who formed the interview sample were unanimously in favour of incorporating such training into community nurse education. Most of the nurses introduced this subject spontaneously when asked about areas of telephone practice that they might like to develop.

The need for self-awareness was the facet of telephone communication skills most frequently discussed. Nurses (CPNs and others) commonly said that they had become sensitized to the subject of telephone manner through overhearing others (often colleagues) speaking on the phone. Several nurses suggested that poor telephone manner is often related to a lack of confidence which may be largely the result of inexperience. The consensus of opinion was that community nurses usually learn by experience and, thus, improve over time. However, the nurses thought that telephone training would be advantageous and three main reasons were given for this:

1. With appropriately timed training, community nurses might become more confident and proficient in telephone skills earlier in their careers. The following words, spoken by a CPN, echo a point made by McDonald (1987): 'it [telephone training] might hasten things on. Experience or experiential learning is extremely important but you can do some of that on people that aren't going to be harmed by your mistakes.'

2. It may be that some nurses do not learn adequately by experience alone and need training to act as a catalyst. Again, an extract from a CPN interview mirrors issues discussed in the literature (Dershewitz, 1980): 'It is something that you learn on your feet with a phone in your hand. But probably everyone doesn't [learn] and that's probably reflected in some people's reluctance to use the phone.'

3. Several nurses (particularly HVs) remarked that even confident and proficient people might gain from telephone training.

The nurses interviewed readily acknowledged the relationship between a good telephone manner and self-awareness. Matters relating to awareness of clients through audible cues (such as sighs and silences) did not, however, emerge quite so spontaneously. This seems important, given that both the postal survey and the interviews identified lack of non-verbal communication as one of the chief perceived difficulties in telephone work. Data from the postal survey reveal that 42% of CPN, 34% of DN and 36% of HV respondents felt this to be a major disadvantage of telephone, as opposed to face-to-face, consultation. For CPNs it was the most frequently cited disadvantage and occupied second place in this respect amongst DNs and HVs. The following comment from a CPN interview illustrates this point:

> I think it is possibly easier to say the negative things about using the phone: you haven't got eye-to-eye contact, you can't observe body language, you can't see and that's a big chunk of communication, isn't it?

One HV thought that the current tendency of communication skills training to concentrate on visual information and non-verbal communication might have the following effect:

> I think that nurses would shy away from using it [the telephone] as a means of counselling because they wouldn't be getting all the cues that they are looking for, or they have been trained to look for.

Although the nurses interviewed have clearly given thought to partially compensating clients for a lack of non-verbal communication (through adoption of an appropriate telephone manner), factors that might mitigate their own difficulties seemed to be less well-conceptualized. A few of the nurses discussed audible cues after some probing and direct questioning. Fairly typically, one CPN when asked about 'a telephone equivalent of non-verbal communication that could be taught' answered 'I think the pitch and tone of voice and the silences – those sort of things'. However, she then went on to say:

> I think it's the responding over the phone that I would perhaps find difficult because I think, personally, I would be checking on whether they were still on the end of the line and, if it was supposed to be a reflective-like silence, interrupting that.

The foregoing remark demonstrates interplay between awareness and self-awareness and suggests that, in some circumstances at least, the latter may be the most troublesome area for community nurses. It is, thus, difficult to determine whether telephone manner, self-awareness and related subjects are mentioned more frequently than audible cues and awareness because they are better conceptualized or because they are more problematic. For this reason, both aspects should be given equal weight when considering appropriate training course content.

While all the nurses interviewed professed that they had gained both confidence and expertise over time (length of time in community practice ranged from 3 to 21 years), certain aspects of telephone work were acknowledged to give rise to feelings of anxiety and inadequacy. The two most commonly mentioned areas were adequate assessment of problems and situations, and dealing with unknown people. A combination of these two factors proves very difficult for some, as the following quotation from a CPN illustrates:

> When we cover for each other when people are on holiday, sometimes the Samaritans get a call from a person who says that they have, or have had, a community psychiatric nurse. On three occasions I have had the Samaritans actually put people through, or I have rung them back in a telephone box and I don't know them from Adam. It is quite frightening in a way, especially when they say 'Well, I am going to do this, I am going to do that'. . . . It is more difficult on the phone, I feel.

Several of the nurses interviewed thought that training might help to increase skills and confidence in these two problem areas. The reference to the Samaritans in the quotation above is interesting, in that this organization was frequently cited as providing a model of good practice for telephone training. The facts that the Samaritans deal with unknown people and are thought to place emphasis on telephone listening skills were seen as relevant in this context. A HV who was considering making herself more accessible to the practice population in general, but who was not totally comfortable about dealing with unknown people over the phone, said the following:

> neither of you know each other and there's just an instrument between you . . . but maybe if you do a course on telephone skills you find it's better than you think. We're getting back to the Samaritans: they must be taught on the same lines to do with counselling skills – where you let the client talk. And if it works well for them, I should imagine that there's something to be learnt. And you do have to listen a lot anyway because, if you're wanting someone to give you a list of symptoms, you've got to ask the question and then give them time to think.

The idea that listening skills, which are more frequently discussed in the context of counselling, are also a key component of assessment skills is made explicit in the above extract.

Several of the nurses interviewed, including CPNs, acknowledged major differences between the work that they do over the phone and that of the Samaritans. The most important of these could be characterized as differences in role, relationship and responsibility. However, as the case of the CPN who received referrals from the Samaritans exemplifies, CPNs in particular are sometimes called upon to deal with similar situations. One CPN said that members of his team frequently dealt with distressed unknown people 'very much on a Samaritans model'.

However, the main issue for nurses was not similarities or differences in work carried out but the transferability of telephone skills taught to Samaritans. Interviewees thought that many of these skills might be useful to community nurses, but tended to have no clear ideas about the specific content of a Samaritan training course, as illustrated by the following comment, made by a CPN: 'I am not sure what sort of training the Samaritans get. I know it is fairly intensive.'

Although many of the nurses interviewed felt that their telephone skills could be improved, unsolicited comments made by respondents to the client survey revealed no dissatisfaction with the nurses' manner or handling of problems over the telephone. It seems likely that the 'telephone-positive' attitude of these particular nurses is reflected in good telephone practice. Whether the telephone work of community nurses in general is viewed favourably by service users remains open to conjecture.

Some nurses may only wish to use the phone for relatively instrumental work, such as appointment-making, which may not require a high degree of skill. However, as one HV pointed out, nurses may need to develop the self-awareness to judge if they are meeting their own needs, rather than those of service users, by automatically dealing with problems face-to-face rather than by telephone. In addition, another HV highlighted what sometimes happens when clients call to request a visit:

> Sometimes people will say 'Could you visit?' And then they'll start – you know, there's a catch in their voice and they're nearly crying and you say something and then they start to talk away. You still visit but you help them at that particular time.

Telephone training may, therefore, enable community nurses to meet the needs of service users: some of those nurses who are reluctant to use the phone for work of an expressive nature might benefit from it most.

SUMMARY

Data from the postal survey suggest that the amount of CPN time spent on telephone work with service users has increased substantially over the last 15 years. However, CPNs receive fewer calls from service users than

HVs and the balance of their telephone work is towards nurse-initiated calls. Although CPNs seem to have slightly better telephone facilities than their DN and HV colleagues, they perhaps employ fewer strategies for ensuring user access. In addition, only 30% of CPN respondents wished to develop their use of telephone consultation. However, no questionnaire items sought views specific to special telephone services or telephone training.

The telephone-positive CPNs interviewed were largely in favour of increasing user access. Some said that, ideally, they would like to run telephone advice lines and duty systems and/or publicize their availability by telephone to the general public. However, there were concerns that such services would be 'swamped' by callers with psychosocial concerns, to the disadvantage of people living with dementia and serious mental health problems (and, perhaps especially, their carers). Many also felt that resources were unlikely to be made available for such schemes. Those wishing to provide this type of service might liaise closely with local voluntary helplines dealing with specific disorders. Where no such helplines exist, CPNs and voluntary agencies might collaborate in relevant pilot schemes.

It is possible that some CPNs are reluctant to develop telephone use because of lack of confidence in a medium which provides no visual information. CPN interviewees pointed out that the Samaritans have a long history of training volunteers to cope with this situation. CPNs who are interested in the subject of telephone training might conduct research to determine the experiences and views of both service users and colleagues.

ACKNOWLEDGEMENTS

This chapter is based on Department of Health funded research and as such is covered by Crown Copyright.

REFERENCES

Angel, S., Nicholl, J. and Amatiello, W. (1988) *Out of Hours. An assessment of the felt and expressed need for an 'out-of-hours' telephone advisory service*, Bristol and Weston Health Authority, Bristol.

Beech, C.P. (1981) A new service for parents with crying babies. *Nursing Times*, **77**, 245–6.

Bryan, J. (1988) Help that is just a phone call away. *The Independent*, **5 Jan**, 12.

Cave, L.A. (1989) Follow-up phone calls after discharge. *American Journal of Nursing*, **89**, 942–3.

Coyne, A.C. (1991) Information and referral service usage among caregivers for dementia patients. *Gerontologist*, **31**, 384–8.

Curtis, P. and Talbot, A. (1981) The telephone in primary care. *Journal of Community Health*, **6**, 194–203.

Davies, P.G.K. (1982) The functioning of British counselling hotlines: a pilot study. *British Journal of Guidance and Counselling*, **10**, 195–9.

Dershewitz, R. (1980) Telephone triage: time for the bell to stop tolling. *Public Health Reports*, **95**, 326–7.

Diseker, R.A., Michielutte, R. and Morrison, V. (1980) Use and reported effectiveness of Tel-med: a telephone health information system. *American Journal of Public Health*, **70**, 229–34.

Drummond, W.J. (1980) Profiles of Youthliners and issues relating to a telephone counselling service in a New Zealand city. *Adolescence*, **15**, 159–70.

Dunnell, K. and Dobbs, J. (1982) *Nurses Working in the Community*, HMSO, London.

Elkins, R.L., Jr. and Cohen, C.R. (1982) A comparison of the effects of prejob training and job experience on nonprofessional telephone crisis counsellors. *Suicide and Life-threatening Behavior*, **12**, 84–9.

Evens, S. and Curtis, P. (1983) Using patient-simulators to teach telephone communication skills to health professionals. *Journal of Medical Education*, **58**, 894–8.

Goodman, H.C. and Perrin, E.C. (1978) Evening telephone call management by nurse practitioners and physicians. *Nursing Research*, **27**, 233–7.

Greenwood, G. (1979) A cry in the night and help is immediate. *Nursing Mirror*, **148**, 24–7.

Hallam, L. (1989) You've got a lot to answer for, Mr Bell: a review of the use of the telephone in primary care. *Family Practice*, **6**, 47–57.

Hampson, S. J. (1989) Nursing interventions for the first three postpartum months. *Journal of Obstetric, Gynaecological and Neonatal Nursing*, **18**, 116–22.

Hirsch, S. (1981) A critique of volunteer-staffed suicide prevention centres. *Canadian Journal of Psychiatry*, **26**, 406–10.

Hornblow, A.R. and Sloane, H.R. (1980) Evaluating the effectiveness of a telephone counselling service. *British Journal of Psychiatry*, **137**, 377–8.

Knowles, D. (1979) On the tendency for volunteer helpers to give advice. *Journal of Counselling Psychology*, **26**, 352–4.

McDonald, G.F. (1987) The simulated clinical laboratory. *Nursing Outlook*, **35**, 290–2.

Munroe, D. and Natale, P. (1982) After-hours call in a primary care nursing practice. *Nurse Practitioner*, **7**, 24–7.

O'Donnell, J.M. and George, K. (1977) The use of volunteers in a community mental health centre emergency and reception service: a comparative study of professional and lay telephone counselling. *Community Mental Health Journal*, **13**, 3–12.

O'Donovan, S. (1993) Call for help. *Nursing Times*, **89**, 30–3.

Parnell, J.W. (1978) *Community Psychiatric Nurses*, Queen's Nursing Institute, London.

Pope, C.R., Yoshioka, S.S. and Greenlick, M.R. (1971) Determinants of medical care: the user of the telephone for reporting symptoms. *Journal of Health and Social Behavior*, **12**, 155–62.

Rainey, L.C. (1985) Cancer counselling by telephone help-line: the UCLA Psychosocial Cancer Counselling Line. *Public Health Reports*, **100**, 308–15.

Rawdon Smith, J. (1984) Introduction of seven day health visiting cover in Peterborough. *Health Visitor*, **57**, 53–4.

Slevin, M.L., Terry, Y., Hallett, N. *et al.* (1988) BACUP – the first two years: evaluation of a national cancer information service. *British Medical Journal*, **297**, 669–72.

Tapp, J.T., Slaikeu, K.A. and Tulkin, S.R. (1974) Toward an evaluation of telephone counselling: process and technical variables influencing 'shows' and 'no-shows' for a clinic referral. *American Journal of Community Psychology*, **2**, 357–64.

Varah, C. (1973) *The Samaritans in the 70s*, Constable, London.

Walfish, S. (1983) Crisis telphone counsellors' views of clinical interaction situations. *Community Mental Health Journal*, **19**, 219–26.

White, E. (1990a) *Community Psychiatry Nursing: The 1990 National Survey*, CPNA Publications, Bradford.

White, E. (1990b) *The National Directory of Community Psychiatric Nursing Services*, CPNA Publications, Bradford.

Wilkinson, G.S., Mirand, E.A. and Graham, S. (1976) Measuring response to a cancer information telephone facility: Can-Dial. *American Journal of Public Health*, **66**, 367–71.

Winogrond, I.R. and Mirassou, M.M. (1983) A crisis intervention service: comparison of younger and older adult clients. *Gerontologist*, **23**, 370–6.

CHAPTER SIX

Project 2000: the early experience of mental health nurses

Edward White

INTRODUCTION

The significance of clinical learning in the preparation of first level nurses has been acknowledged for many years. However, a literature has accumulated over more than a decade which has demonstrated the complexity of providing a good learning experience (Alexander, 1983). The role played by practitioners and the environment in which student learning takes place have both been identified as being particularly significant (Pembrey, 1980; Ogier, 1982; Reid, 1985; Jacka and Lewin, 1987; Hyland, Millard and Parker, 1988; Ryan, 1989; Marriott, 1991).

Prior to the introduction of Project 2000 (United Kingdom Central Council, 1986), an early experience of which provided the context for the present study, an apprenticeship model was predominant in nurse education. This model, which required students to meet the demands of service as well as their own educational needs, had received extensive criticism, not only in nursing but also within other areas of professional education (Jarvis, 1983). Thus, as new goals and aspirations have been articulated for nursing practice within new-style arrangements for service provision, it has behoved nurse educationalists to design Project 2000 (P2K) course curricula that fulfil these new requirements.

This has created a new set of major challenges. For example, it has been necessary to make arrangements to prepare students of nursing to work in both institutional and community settings and then to locate appropriate practice settings for students to achieve the learning objectives. Moreover, the demand for collaboration with institutions of higher education, in order to prepare students for qualification which has both academic and professional currency, has led educationalists to a rethink of not only the theoretical components of the course, but also the practical dimension. In particular, the level of practice to be demonstrated by the student has had to be reconsidered and engaged as part of the new course validation process (While, 1991).

The demands that these changes will make on practitioners in the future were recognized both by the United Kingdom Central Council for Nursing, Midwifery and Health Visiting (UKCC) and the English National Board for Nursing, Midwifery and Health Visiting (ENB). Indeed, the UKCC has clearly acknowledged the need for appropriate preparation for practitioners to fulfil their changed role, while the ENB has developed this aspect further and raised questions about the assignment of appropriate roles and titles to those practitioners involved in student learning. Similarly, the introduction of super-numerary status within P2K , although not a new concept in nurse education, has not generally been applied outside undergraduate programmes. Here, the complexities of the process, particularly in acknowledging the changing needs of students as they progress through the course, have long been acknowledged. So, too, the difficulties of integrating theory and practice have also previously been demonstrated (Bendall, 1975; Clarke, 1986; McCaugherty, 1991).

These issues confirm the complexity of clinical supervision (Fish and Purr, 1991; Butterworth and Faugier, 1992) and have raised questions about the different roles played by individual practitioners. Thus, although learning through practice has been regarded as fundamental to effective professional education and the development of competence in clinical practice, the extent to which this process is currently overcoming the theory/practice gap in Project 2000 nurse education has remained questionable. Indeed, more than a decade ago, Merriam (1983) reviewed the literature across several disciplines for common findings, trends or generalizations, but had to conclude that it was very difficult to work out exactly how important mentors were. Despite this, as Burnard (1988) more recently noted, the term 'mentorship' seemed to have 'slipped into the folklore of nurse education almost unnoticed and quickly became part of the educational language of the eighties and nineties'.

It was against such a controversial backdrop that the present study was commissioned and undertaken. The present writer was the full-time principal researcher to the research study. With the commitment of a full-time research assistant (Elizabeth Riley) and part-time assistance provided by two teaching colleagues (Susan Davies and Sheila Twinn), whose contributions are readily acknowledged here, a detailed study was conducted into aspects of both adult and mental health nursing education (White *et al.*, 1994).

While the completed study found that most of the substantive issues were applicable to both branches, this chapter will concentrate on mental health nursing perspective (in hospital and community settings), for which the writer held sole responsibility. Moreover, although the recent report of the Mental Health Nursing Review Team recognized 'the importance of the historic development of community psychiatric nursing services and the part they played in developing the profession and changing services', the Review Team believed that 'the continued separation between community and inpatient nursing militated against continuity of care' (Department of Health, 1994). Indeed, the Team suggested 'avoidance of terminology which discriminated between nurses working in community and inpatient settings'. Evidence to this effect has already been witnessed by the recent change of name to the erstwhile *Community Psychiatric Nursing Journal* which has become *Mental Health Nursing*; still the journal of the Community Psychiatric Nurses Association. Thus, findings reported here will draw upon sources of data from community and inpatient domains, not only to reflect the change to the nomenclature but rather to confirm the commonality of the issues found for mental health nurses in both settings.

In October 1990, the ENB put out to tender a project specification for a 2-year research study of the relationships between teaching, support, supervision and role modelling for students in clinical areas within the context of Project 2000 courses. The ENB believed that all these activities were important in the learning process, but was concerned that 'it could not be presumed that the present arrangements were ideal or the most appropriate, or that, for example, mentorship was necessarily the best way to provide elements of support and role modelling'. The ENB required the commissioned study to provide answers to the issue of the effectiveness of the prevailing circumstance and to indicate whether changes were needed.

The project specification required the study to focus on the latter half of first-wave Project 2000 demonstration courses, to account for the different specialist clinical areas in the branch programmes. Moreover, the study was to include attention to:

1. the interrelationships of the different roles for the provision of teaching, support, supervision and role modelling;
2. the merits and demerits of distinguishing the roles in principle and in practice;
3. the nature and variability of the mentor role in current practice;
4. models of good practice for student teaching, support, supervision and role modelling;
5. alternative arrangements for more effective teaching, support, supervision and role modelling;
6. identification of the personnel who should occupy the roles;
7. the preparation required for the roles.

In order to operationalize these interests, a study was designed which examined the relationships between the different roles which were pre-specified by the ENB, by directing a focus upon individuals who occupied such roles *in vivo*. Thus, an interest in the relationship between, say, teaching and supervision, was translated into an empirical examination of the real life relationships between teachers and supervisors.

AIMS

Accordingly, the following set of aims was agreed for the present study, which could be accommodated within the time, expertise and budget available:

1. to analyse the concepts of teacher, supporter, mentor and supervisor, both in the literature and as seen by those individuals involved in facilitating clinical learning;
2. to explore the perceptions and interpretations of the value of these roles, by those involved in the adult and mental health branch programmes of Project 2000 courses;
3. to make recommendations about the appropriate preparation for practitioners undertaking such roles in the clinical learning environment.

METHODOLOGY

Having been scrutinized and accepted by responsible officers of the ENB during the application process for funding, the methodology and data collection methods were also subsequently accepted by the ENB-approved Steering Group. The Steering Group comprised 10 individuals with both national and international reputations in nursing and/or education and/or research, who were drawn from different English universities and colleges, the National Foundation for Educational Research and the National Health Service Management Executive/Department of Health. The purpose of this group was to provide the research team with an independent steer to ensure rigorous thinking on the methodological issues, not only as they emerged during the 2 years of the study but also as they were reported in the full, final report submitted to the commissioning agency. Their guidance and support is readily acknowledged here.

As many of the central research questions and interests were complex and contentious (a clear impression confirmed by the review of the literature), an interactive approach was favoured. A qualitative field study (Fielding and Fielding, 1986; Lofland and Lofland, 1984) was thus agreed. A case methodology (Yin, 1984) provided an opportunity to try to understand the experience of those directly connected with student learning and to focus on direct, face-to-face knowledge of their circumstance in natural social settings. Appropriate data collection methods were decided to include tape-recorded interviews, non-participant observation and documentary evidence.

The study was therefore designed to satisfactorily address the three aims, which themselves operationalized the seven areas of interest of the ENB.

Table 6.1 Overview of study design

Preliminary investigations
Focused interviews with key figures in nurse education
Scrutiny of P2K course submission documents
Self-completion questionnaire to college principals

Stage 1
Semi-structured interviews in three centres with:

Mental Health Branch	*Adult Branch*
Students ($n = 23$)	Students ($n = 30$)
Practitioners ($n = 20$)	Practitioners ($n = 17$)
Tutors ($n = 8$)	Tutors ($n = 17$)

Stage 2
Six case studies:

Mental Health Branch	*Adult Branch*
Three case studies (one in each of three centres)	Three case studies (one in each of three centres)

Each case study consisted of three separate practice settings, in each of which observation, interviews and documentary evidence were used to collect information

---

From an overview of the methodology (Table 6.1) it can be seen that, following preparatory work, a two-stage study was designed.

Preliminary investigations

A wide-ranging preparatory interview was undertaken with experts in nurse education, as a means to explore the context within which the study was to take place and to become familiar with the width of issues involved.

Having sought and received written permission from the appropriate institutions, all 42 Project 2000 course submission documents which had been received by the ENB for validation purposes were scrutinized in-house. The examination of these documents focused upon the way in which roles had been identified to facilitate student learning in practice settings and upon the titles assigned to these roles.

A follow-up survey (see Marsh, 1982 for exemplar methodological advice) was then undertaken, in which the principals of all 42 institutions were contacted in writing. Each respondent was invited to confirm the titles used in their local centres to identify the roles occupied by the practitioners and tutors who were formally instrumental in helping Project 2000 students to learn in practical placement areas of the Adult and Mental Health Branch Programmes. In addition, the principals were invited to identify the functions performed by the holders of each title. The purpose of this enquiry was to gain an indication of the properties of all the roles identified and to better understand the dimensional ranges of commonly used terms.

Stage 1

In April 1991, when work on this study began, 13 centres in England had commenced Project 2000 courses and thus formed the only sampling frame available. Six of these were the focus of a Government-funded study undertaken by the National Foundation for Educational Research (NFER), which aimed at a broader evaluation of the implementation of Project 2000. These centres were automatically exluded from the options available, in order to avoid the problem of over-researching. The remaining seven centres were approached to establish their willingness to participate in the present research. One centre declined because of ongoing local research, while another centre (also the focus of a local evaluation) declined to participate in the main study, but offered to make themselves available for pilot work. This centre was involved in the pilot of Stage 1 research instruments. The remaining five all expressed a willingness to be fully involved. The three colleges furthest into the branch programme at the time when data were to be collected (and thus with the most experience to recount) were finally selected as the main study centres. One of the two that remained was selected for Stage 2 pilot work. All three main study centres were in the south of England and were respectively located in rural, urban and inner city areas.

In order to identify and explore the issues most pertinent to student learning in practice settings, it was essential to capture the views and experiences of the key actors, by which was meant the students, the tutorial staff and the clinical practitioners. This triangulation of respondents allowed the perspectives of the main participants in student learning to be compared and any ambiguity and potential conflict within roles to be highlighted. Focused, semi-structured interviews were considered an appropriate vehicle by which to explore an understanding and interpretation of the key terms that appeared to occur in both branches. A list of themes and issues were identified which had emerged from the literature and from the preliminary investigations and broad topic areas were translated into specific questions, which were then refined. Two separate interview schedules were produced, one for tutors and clinical practitioners and one for students. In common with that designed for students, the qualified staff schedule included items which attempted to locate and explore models of good practice, from which lessons could be learnt. Each was piloted in two non-participating centres, one in the north of England, the other in the east, and minor alterations were made as a consequence.

Written approval was sought and obtained from local health authority research ethics committees in each of the pilot and main study centres.

In each centre, an introductory visit was arranged for members of the research team to share information about the project and make the logistical arrangements for data collection. A wide range of people were invited to attend, including the college principals, course leaders, branch leaders (from both mental health and adult), practitioner representatives from both institutional and community placement areas and student representatives. These meetings proved worthwhile in the dissemination of information about the proposed research and in making contact with potential respondents, as those present were usually the conduit by which appropriate tutors and service staff could be approached for interview. Separate meetings were arranged with student groups, to explain the aims and methods of the research and to request volunteers for interview. A written abstract of the research aims and study design was widely disseminated within the study centres.

Purposive samples were drawn of tutors, practitioners and students ($n = 115$) in the three main study centres, of which 51 were concerned with mental health. Care was taken to reflect the characteristics of age, gender and ethnicity of the group as a whole and, in the case of students, a spectrum of opinion regarding their experience of the course (Table 6.2).

Interviews were conducted in each centre over a 3-week period and started with the centre that was furthest into its course. Verbal consent was obtained from all participants and tapes and data sheets were coded to protect anonymity. The researchers gave an undertaking to ensure that individual respondents' identities would be rendered anonymous in written reports. Information about a respondent's age and ethnicity was elicited by the use of prompt cards. The interview schedules were used as a guide, to ensure that all topics were covered, but ample scope was also provided to explore unpredictable areas of interest in more detail. Each interview lasted between 30 and 90 minutes and was tape-recorded.

Data analysis proceeded concurrently with data collection, on the basis of typescripts produced from a verbatim transcription of the interview tapes (see Appendix for an example). It became apparent, however, that the themes which emerged from each group of respondents (students, practitioners, tutors) quickly approached saturation and the necessity for the further transcription of all interview audiotapes for the sequential analysis to continue was questioned. The ratio of interview length to transcription time ranged between 1:4 and 1:6. That is, 1 hour of audiotape took an agency typist about 4–6 hours to transcribe; there was, therefore, an important financial dimension to this activity. It was considered that no advantage had been conferred on the analytic process by working on data available in a conventional typescript format. Moreover, it was felt that the methodological rigour of the analysis would not be compromised if it proceeded on the basis of actual audiotaped data replayed by the researchers (the equivalent of a re-read of the tyepscript). Indeed, on balance, it was felt that the richness of the data was more likely to be appreciated when heard than when read. Advice on this matter was

Table 6.2 Summary of characteristics of Stage 1 respondents (M = male; F = female; * = missing data)

	Sex		Age (years)									Ethnicity	
	M	F	18–23	24–29	30–34	35–39	40–44	45–49	50–54	55+	*	White	Other
Students	25	28	24	17	6	5	1	0	0	0	0	48	5
Adult Branch	9	21	20	4	2	3	1	0	0	0	0	28	2
Mental Health Branch	16	7	4	13	4	2	0	0	0	0	0	20	3
Practitioners	9	28	0	9	10	6	9	0	0	1	2	32	5
Adult Branch	1	16	0	4	4	3	3	0	0	1	2	17	0
Mental Health Branch	8	12	0	5	6	3	6	0	0	0	0	15	5
Tutors	8	17	0	4	5	8	4	2	1	1	0	21	4
Adult Branch	1	16	0	4	5	4	3	0	0	1	0	17	0
Mental Health Branch	7	1	0	0	0	4	1	2	1	0	0	4	4
Totals	42	73	24	30	21	19	14	2	1	2	2	101	14

sought from academic researchers, within and beyond the Steering Group and, as a result, a decision was taken to limit the transcriptions to approximately one-third of the tapes, chosen purposively. These transcriptions were then used as an adjunct when actual tape-recordings were listened to and analysed by the researchers. The tape-recorded interviews for which a full verbatim transcript was not produced had telling fragments summarized and tagged (by means of the counter number on the tape-recorder) for later possible verbatim transcription for inclusion in this report. This methodological adjustment was found to work very well in practice.

In order to organize these fragments of data in a coherent fashion, an A3-size matrix was constructed with the categories from the content analysis on the *y* axis and individual respondents on the *x* axis. Three of these matrices were made for each branch: one each for the students, practitioners and tutors data. This structure of empty cells thus handled the products derived from a content analysis (Holsti, 1969) of the interview data. This involved the extraction of telling fragments of data from each interview which could be located in a relevant cell. Issues that emerged which did not fit into an established category were added to the axis to approximate categories which were, as far as could be handled practically, mutually exclusive and exhaustive. Such a method allowed a comparison to be made between respondent groups and between branches, settings and centres.

Stage 2

In order to explore and develop a deeper understanding of the issues emerging from Stage 1 interview data, case studies were undertaken as the basis of the second stage of data collection. Case study is a research strategy that can be likened to an experiment, a history or a simulation, which may be considered alternative research strategies. None of these are linked to a particular type of evidence or method of data collection. As a research strategy, the distinguishing characteristic of the case study is that it attempts to examine:

1. a contemporary phenomenon in its real life context; especially when,
2. the boundaries between phenomenon and context are not clearly evident.

Experiments differ from this in that they deliberately divorce a phenomenon from its context. Histories differ in that they are limited to past phenomena, where relevant informants may be unavailable for interview and relevant events unavailable for direct observation (Yin, 981). This was therefore a highly appropriate method for the present study to adopt, as it focused on the 'lived' experiences of those undergoing change and so specifically addressed the interests of the ENB.

In the present study, six case studies were undertaken. Three were devoted to the Adult Branch and three to the Mental Health Branch. One of each took place in three separate centres in England. Data were captured from three different settings in each case study. For the Mental Health Branch, this meant two were planned in the community and one in hospital.

Settings were selected within the three centres, according to the following criteria:

1. that students would be available in particular settings during the time window for data collection;
2. that students, clinical and tutorial staff were willing to participate in the work.

It was initially expected that the selection of the case study settings would be able to satisfy a third criterion: that, as a result of a consensus amongst Stage 1 respondents, a particular setting was viewed as a positive learning environment for Project 2000 students (a so-called 'good model'). However, in the event, it was found that such consensus between respondents did not exist. Moreover, respondents often hesitated and/or offered caveats before they committed themselves to identify any setting as a good model of practice for student teaching, support, supervision and role modelling. This feature occurred at all three centres and meant that one of the pre-specified interests of the ENB would prove very difficult to satisfy.

The main methods of data collection employed within each case study included non-participant observation, tape-recorded periods of actual interaction and semi-structured interviews. The main focus for data collection was the students' learning experiences during pre-specified work periods. In order to gain an insight into the processes involved in their clinical learning, students were observed during two working days (often traditional shifts) on two separate occasions. The role adopted by each researcher during these periods accorded with the conventional notion of 'observer as participant' (Polgar and Thomas, 1988).

The number of hours spent by researchers in non-participant observation in the Adult Branch was 118 hours. For the Mental Health Branch, in which one centre had abandoned the traditional student 'placement' arrangement in favour of a client allocation model and in another access to observation in community settings was denied, periods of non-participant observation amounted to 70 hours. Thus, the total amounted to approximately 188 hours of observation, shared between the remaining two full-time researchers (EW and ER) and one part-timer (SD). The second part-time colleague (ST) had emigrated halfway through the study and was not replaced.

Each period of observation was followed by a separate debriefing interview both with the student and with the main person identified as helping them learn within the practice setting. Insight into aspects of organization such as role differentiation, teaching strategies and the student's consequent experience was developed by means of in-depth interviews with other key pesonnel involved in facilitating the student's learning. Data derived from these data collection methods again addressed all the ENB interests and all the aims. A profile was developed for each setting, from data derived from a structured questionnaire and separate documentary sources.

Verbal consent was obtained from student and practitioner respondents prior to the commencement of fieldwork in each setting and immediately prior to each period of observation and interview. At the beginning of each 'shift' of observation in a ward setting, the researcher introduced her/himself to patients likely to be involved in observation/tape-recording and gave a brief outline of the study. Verbal consent to participation in the study was sought from all patients in both institutional and community settings. All tapes and field notes were coded to protect anonymity.

Methodological critique. The notion of representativeness was neither possible nor sought. Rather, the samples owed their selection to the twin notions of opportunity and quota; indeed, this was the only practical way to have proceeded. It is nevertheless acknowledged here as a limitation to the study, imposed by the parameters of the method, in which (to use the words of Yates, cited in Moser and Stuart, 1953) 'the researcher is continually looking over his shoulder and wondering whether some extraneous factor exists which will vitiate the conclusions based on his conclusions'. However, it is also recognized here that **all** research is limited by methodological constraints and that all social researchers, quite independent of paradigm, are not (and should not ever be) absolutely free of such doubt. An appropriate analogy has been reported by Yin (1981):

> There are no fixed recipes for building, or comparing explanations. An analogous situation may be found in doing detective work, where a detective must construct an explanation for the crime. Presented with the scene of the crime, its description and possible reports from eye witnesses, the detective must constantly make decisions regarding the relevance of various data. Some facts of the case will turn out to be unrelated to the crime; other clues must be recognized as such and pursued vigorously. The adequate explanation for the crime then becomes a plausible rendition of a motive, opportunity and method that more fully accounts for the facts than do alternative explanations.

Part of the explicit purpose for the present study was to make available in the public domain examples of different practices that would lend themselves to scrutiny and to being judged for their relevance in local settings. Thus, the research team closely monitored the themes that emerged from the accounts provided by other investigators (see, for examples, Jowett, Walton and Payne, 1992; Orton, Prowse and Millen, 1993) who had conducted similar research simultaneously in different fieldwork settings, looking for areas of commonality with findings presented here; most of the findings were apparent in other research. Moreover, papers given by the present writer at several conferences in England since the study has been completed, including one dedicated to the findings at the International Congress on Mental Health Nursing at the University of Manchester Institute of Science and Technology and another dedicated to the methodology at the Royal College of Nursing Annual Research Conference at the University of Glasgow, have served to support the credentials of both. Thus, while a claim of representativeness was methodologically inappropriate, the contention is that the insights derived from this carefully conducted study, addressing the pre-specified research interests of the English National Board and the aims of the study, are unlikely to be rogue or without popular currency, and will have a resonance and practical utility to a wide audience beyond the study centres.

FINDINGS

Mental Health Branch students across all centres criticized the content of the Common Foundation Programmes (CFP) for being unacceptably biased toward 'general' nursing and, whereas the Adult Branch was seen (but here only in a relative sense) as a seamless continuation of the CFP, the Mental Health Branch was not. Most Mental Health Branch students felt their course only really began a year and a half after it had nominally started.

> I felt that the course hadn't prepared me at all for Mental Health. It was a view being voiced by a number of students. I think it was because of the General bias in the CFP, because most of the people who taught us in the CFP were General tutors. I think this is where it came from. Because of the way I was feeling, I actually said 'I want out. This is my career I am talking about. I want to switch.' I was actually told that there was no position in the General (Adult) branch. So I either did the Psychiatric, or I left the course. (Student, Mental Health Branch)

> We've lost out; because we've got to start now [in the Mental Health Branch]. Whereas the others [Adult Branch students] will have had three years General training. (Student, Mental Health Branch)

> What happens with them, is that students come into the block at the start of the Branch and what we try to do is to give them RMN training in 18 months. As far as I can see, we're trying to ram everything that we would have given them [RMN students] into 18 months. (Tutor, Mental Health)

One of the issues this created for the qualified nurses (the practitioners) who were charged with the responsibility to help Mental Health Branch students learn in practice settings was characterized by the sentiment 'we now have to do more, because they have done less'. On occasion, the additional demands posed by Project 2000 students had already reached breaking point, because not only had the nature of the demand changed, but so too had the relentlessness of the pressure: 'too many students and not enough placements', as it was put.

One community psychiatric nurse respondent had considered falling back on the UKCC Code of Conduct, because student placements had begun to compromise the quality of her clinical practice and that of her colleagues who were in the same position. As she put it:

> The Project 2000 student I've got is more demanding of me. Wanting me to help him with some project he's doing on schizophrenia. But he doesn't know anything about schizophrenia. So it's starting from scratch and that is very, very draining. You're driving along in the car, talking about schizophrenia and he's saying 'that's very, very interesting' and taking notes down. I've not experienced that before. It feels as if I'm doing a lecture, from one client to the next. There's absolutely no time for me to reflect on what I'm doing and how I'm working with the clients, because so much is being taken out of me by the student.
>
> (Community Psychiatric Nurse)

Some 200 miles away from that CPN, in a different centre, senior nursing staff had already declined a request to allocate additional Project 2000 students to a busy hospital ward, on the grounds that it would put at risk the quality of patient care. In the third centre, a D-graded hospital-based mental health nurse reported similar sentiments about the constant pressure involved in supervising Project 2000 Branch students. This was especially so when (as was the case when our fieldwork was undertaken) she was the only qualified member of nursing staff on duty, supported by two young nursing assistants. Although she was only 7 months out of RMN training herself, she had sole responsibility for the care of 23 acute psychiatric admission patients. Of her Project 2000 student, she reported:

> I think 'just go away and leave me alone'. I have to try and quell my irritation and maybe send her [Project 2000 student] off on an errand or something, just to give me 5 minutes breathing space, before I blow my top.
>
> (Staff Nurse, Mental Health)

Mental Health Branch students often worked alone and unsupervised for much of their time, which (in terms of a methodological retrospective) meant that periods of non-participant observation by researchers of head-to-head learning opportunities with qualified nursing staff was akin to 'panning for gold'. Such loneliness was reported particularly by students at one centre, who were subject to an unconventional, context-free, client-allocation model of practical experience, rather than the more usual placement area arrangement. Such an innovation was universally reported by all those connected with it to be very difficult to administer.

Mental health students complained of short and discontinuous placement periods which, when combined with sickness and holidays, meant that student/practitioner contact was often infrequent and superficial. For town-based students who were dependent on public transport, the increasingly federal nature of contemporary community mental health services meant that this was exacerbated by the considerable time, energy and money spent in travelling to the more remote rural areas to secure practical learning experience. That students should spend considerably more uninterrupted time in mental health practice settings was the universal opinion.

> They are shoved from pillar to post, in very short placements. They are never given the time to become a member of a team. They never belong anywhere. So I think they feel quite isolated. A lot of them are probably very scared and quite anxious. I never really get time to settle and resolve all those issues. (Tutor, Mental Health)

With limited opportunities to practise and a lack of relevant and timely theoretical insights gained in the colleges to reflect on and test out *in vivo*, mental health students expressed apprehension about their comparatively low level of skill development. One student likened her experience of the Mental Health Branch to 'being dropped from a plane in France'. During a period of non-participant observation another student was overheard to lament:

> **Third-year Student (Mental Health Branch)**: I am not convinced that the training I've had will equip me to work in the community; not even in hospital.
> **CPN Team Leader**: That's because they've got it wrong with you.

Concomitantly, the lack of educational preparation for mental health practitioners was widely regarded as a 'vital bone of contention' and was apparent in the methods they adopted to facilitate student learning in practice settings, which were frequently task-orientated and not client-centred or relevant to student learning objectives. It largely fell to the students, therefore, to prepare the qualified staff in practice areas, rather than the conventional other way round. In such circumstances, combined with a lack of coordinated contact between practitioners and mental health tutors, the task of making connections between theory and practice was formidable.

There were widespread problems regarding communication about the Project 2000 courses: that is, the relevant information did not get to all the people who needed to know, and a circle of uncertainty resulted. As a consequence, a mismatch of expectation between different role players was common. The roles played by practitioners to help with student learning varied within and between settings. These multifarious roles were not uniformly understood, nor were they tidily enacted, nor were they occupied independent of other competing demands and interests.

Indeed, results from the survey of college principals who, in 1991, intended to host a Project 2000 course (the results of which were later confirmed by data derived from interview and observation) showed that role titles and role functions were entirely interchangeable. None of the different functions was uniquely identified with any of the reported role titles. That is to say, assessors did more than assess; some supervised. Supervisors did more than supervise; some assessed; others mentored. Mentors not only mentored; some supervised; yet others assessed. The interrelationships between the different roles for the provision of teaching, support, supervision and role modelling were thus bereft of distinguishable patterns; a semantic maelstrom.

Some practitioners did not know which role they occupied in relation to student learning; indeed, on occasion, this was disregarded as completely irrelevant. It was not uncommon for practitioners to report that they did exactly the same thing with Project 2000 students as they had previously done with Registered Mental Nurse students. Such a position was defended by one practitioner thus:

> What I do with Project 2000 students isn't any different to what I would do with 'a student'. What I have got to offer hasn't changed, is what I'm saying. My job hasn't changed, so what I have to offer hasn't changed.
>
> (Charge Nurse, Mental Health)

The assessment of Mental Health Branch students' practice was problematic and the instruments for doing so were ambiguous and open to considerable subjective variation. Students in one centre, all holders of first degrees, avoided falling prey to what was universally regarded by them as an 'enormous lottery' by identifying themselves with the 'right' practitioner to assess their practice. As one mental health student put it:

> So far, I've been fortunate enough to find 'soft touches' [to assess me]. That's not for the long-term benefit of my educational development on the course. But it is definitely worth finding somebody who understands the limitations of the course and is prepared to compensate for that.
>
> (Student, Mental Health Branch)

Tutorial staff played an insignificant role in the assessment of practice and scarcely any clinical teaching or intentional role-modelling was either reported or observed by researchers.

Tutors were often overwhelmed by multiple, and sometimes competing, demands on their time and energy. Some tutors reported not having taught at DipHE level before and, on occasion (like some practitioners), not having been prepared themselves to diploma level. It was not rare to find, therefore, that these competing interests were in addition to the demands of their own educational preparation to a higher level.

With little opportunity to visit practice areas, and with Project 2000 students yet to consolidate a confident position, tutors struggled to establish a new identity and an appropriate role within the context of the new course arrangements. Most occupied a troubleshooter's role, which was often focused on general misunderstandings of the assessment process and student learning objectives. Tripartite meetings held in practice areas between students, practitioners and tutors were as welcome as they were rare.

Overall, the notion of diploma level practice and its assessment was very poorly understood by practitioners, tutors and students. Widespread uncertainty, and even unselfconscious ignorance, was reported.

> I don't know what that [Diploma level] is. I mean, how should I know? I know that it is pitched at a higher level than the training that I did. I know it's pitched at a higher level when training the learners, the RMN learners, that are currently going through. I know that they are doing a different syllabus from the syllabus that I did. So, given all these differences, I don't know for example what ultimately is expected of them at diploma level. No, I don't. I don't at all.   (Charge Nurse, Mental Health)

Despite recent confirmation from the English National Board about 'how important it was to realize that a DipHE was not just more of the same as the existing first level courses, but required a fresh approach consonant with a higher education award', this had yet to penetrate the working reality of most of those with their feet on the ground, either in the colleges or in the field.

Although the ENB 998 course (Teaching and Assessing in Clinical Areas) was often innocently thought of as the course of choice, confidence in it as being helpful in this regard was not widespread, not least because of the apparent variation of orientation and quality between different ENB 998 course centres. However, a more appropriate preparation for practitioners was poorly articulated by them; they didn't know what they didn't know.

The notion of supernumerary status was understood and interpreted in different ways and not always wholly embraced by practitioners, especially when staffing levels were low and, on occasion, reported as 'dangerous'. In such circumstances their supernumerary status was compromised into a state virtually indistinguishable from that of rostered service. Generally, supernumerary status meant that students could not be counted on to provide a predictable contribution to service provision; the corollary, however, was that qualified nursing staff could not always be counted on to provide predictable educational support to students. This, because patients always came first; an understandable reality, although one with unsatisfactory outcomes for all concerned with student learning in practice areas.

> The students look to the practitioners [for help]; the practitioners look to the tutors and the tutors are looking for someone themselves. It's a dilemma.
> (Tutor, Mental Health)

Although a rare finding in the present study, models of good practice for student teaching, support, supervision and role modelling were found. This was particularly so in one mental health setting, where qualified nursing staff had the benefit themselves of supernumerary days and therefore had sufficient time to concentrate on educational matters. As the practitioner who had lead responsibility for Project 2000 students in this setting (though he was rarely a mentor, or supervisor, or whatever) put it:

> I think we [the team] transmit the ambience and philosophy of our ward with consummate ease, enthusiasm and commitment and I think it's that which infects them [the students], which is why we are successful. And that is supported by formal academic input.
>
> I think that is what we do best and I think that is why the students like it here. It is really important, no matter what anybody says, that students aren't going to learn unless they like it somewhere
>
> (Charge Nurse, Mental Health)

Students were observed to thrive in this setting, because they were given practical responsibility, in real time, under close and continuous supervision. Debriefing, in particular, through reflection upon actual clinical experiences was universally welcomed by students, independent of context. All students who worked in close collaboration with well-motivated, articulate, fully informed, enthusiastic, qualified staff, reported that they benefited hugely from so doing. Similarly, practitioners were often triggered into a positive mode by the Project 2000 students themselves, who either initiated or reciprocated an enthusiasm to learn.

In the three demonstration course centres used in the present study, overtly positive experiences were rare. In large measure, respondents attributed this dearth to the unpreparedness of practitioners and tutorial staff to accommodate Project 2000 students. This, in turn, was thought to have been the consequence of the unrealistically short timescale for the introduction of Project 2000 in England. At one centre, ENB approval was met with incredulity:

> It would have been helpful to have stopped taking basic [RMN] students, to start taking a serious look at what we were going to do, why we were going to do it and what people's roles would be. We needed time to breathe, instead of getting what I think is a Mickey Mouse curriculum together, which was really thrown together really rapidly. I'm amazed it [Project 2000 course] got approval. I can remember the day before it had to go up for approval, being in this room here with bits of paper on the floor, re-writing objectives and trying to consolidate our objectives to bring the numbers down. It was like a circus here, and nobody really believed that it would possibly be accepted. And it was. I don't believe it.
>
> (Tutor, Mental Health)

CONCLUSION

The implications for mental health nursing *per se*, which the findings from this study have revealed, can be characterized in two ways: those factors which facilitated good learning experience in practice settings for Project 2000 students and those which acted as a barrier to its achievement. Successful facilitation was made possible through fieldwork staff who were committed to teaching students and, in all senses of the term, had the capacity so to do. Such staff were knowledgeable about the educational requirements, felt ownership of the new curriculum and ensured that students were intentionally exposed to well-planned learning experiences. Easy staff relationships and good contact with tutorial staff were hallmarks of this endeavour. The antithesis, however, produced evidence of the barriers to good learning experience: low staffing levels, poor climate and organization of work, weak communication at all levels, staff who lacked the capacity to be motivated and felt unprepared for the student-centred dimension to their jobs.

It is not yet known whether students who have been educationally prepared for work as nurses under Project 2000 will exhibit the expected competencies for work inside the remaining psychiatric hospitals and/or community mental health settings. Neither is it yet known whether the investment in this scheme will yield, or will be likely to yield, a pay-off to the National Health Service. Until compelling evidence for this can be provided, on the basis of discrete empirical research reported here, some confusion and misunderstanding of roles between Project 2000 students, practitioners and tutors has been revealed. These undoubtedly difficult issues, all of which have a bearing on the notion of clinical supervision of Project 2000 students in mental health settings, both inside hospital and in the community, were themselves regarded by key players in one of two different ways. Either they were a temporary consequence of the newness of Project 2000 which would resolve over time or an enduring consequence of an educational arrangement that was flawed at a conceptual level.

Thus, if mental health nursing is to retain speciality at initial preparation level, the rigorous debate ahead in relation to Project 2000 will make matters of curriculum structure and educational process inescapable. So, too, a fundamental consideration of whether 'mental health nursing in the community' is the same as, or different from, 'community mental health nursing'.

APPENDIX

Fragment of verbatim transcript of an interview between the writer (EW) and a mental health nurse tutor.

Interviewer: So; do you have responsibilities for assessing Project 2000 students in clinical areas?

Respondent: No, I haven't. I have taken part in discussion when the mentors were looking at the first assessment. Because they were just starting the mental health branch, there was a new assessment tool; we used Bondy, well, it's an adapted version of the Bondy tool. And was fairly . . . just sort of, helping the student to self-assess themselves. Well where am I in this particular thing? For example, there were things like in the communication skills, which was broken down into several sectors and basically help them to reflect, and to see where they're at, and at what point they are in that particular skill. Because there are five levels, from independent to dependent. So it's really sort of helping them to sort out at what level . . . but the final assessment, no, I haven't been involved.

Interviewer: Right. So; if you don't do it, who does?

Respondent: Well, they have a mentor, a chosen mentor, on the ward, who the bulk of the time they'll be working with. So that their supervisor will have a pretty good idea about where they're at, at this particular time.

Interviewer: Two things, there. First, you said that they were chosen, what do you mean by that? Do you mean that students choose their mentor, or are they simply allocated?

Respondent: They're allocated, yes.

Interviewer: Second thing you said was 'supervisor'.

Respondent: Right.

Interviewer: Did you mean 'supervisor', or 'mentor'?

Respondent: Mentor.

Interviewer: I just wondered if there was another group of people called 'supervisors'.

Respondent: No. No, the same person who is the mentor, but also supervisor. And also could be an assessor [laughs].

Interviewer: Right, we'll unpack it as we go along.

Respondent: Right.

Interviewer: So, you don't have a formal role in assessing Project 2000 students.

Respondent: No.

Interviewer: Right. Is this an appropriate state of affairs, do you think?

Respondent: Er, I think so. Because I think it would be unfair for me to go on the wards and having, not worked for a length of time with the student, to be there and just to go in and assess them. I don't think it's fair. I think one needs to be working with them for a good length of time, before one can actually, honestly, assess them.

ACKNOWLEDGEMENTS

Singular thanks are due to Professor Tony Butterworth for his understanding, advice and rock-solid support.

REFERENCES

Alexander, M. (1983) *Learning to Nurse; Integrating Theory and Practice*, Churchill Livingstone, Edinburgh.

Bendall, E. (1975) *So You Passed Nurse*, Royal College of Nursing, London.

Burnard, P. (1988) Mentors: a supporting act. *Nursing Times*, **84**, 627–8.

Butterworth, T. and Faugier, J. (eds) (1992) *Clinical Supervision and Mentorship in Nursing*, Chapman & Hall, London.

Clarke, M. (1986) Action and reflection: practice and theory in nursing. *Journal of Advanced Nursing*, **1**, 11–13.

Department of Health (1994) *Working in Partnership: a Collaborative Approach to Care*, Report of the Mental Health Nursing Review Team, HMSO, London.

Fielding, N. and Fielding, J. (1986) *Linking Data*, Sage Publications, London.

Fish, D. and Purr, B. (1991) *An Evaluation of Practice Based Learning in Continuing Professional Education, Project Paper 4*, English National Board, London.

Holsti, O. (1969) *Content Analysis for the Social Sciences and Humanities*, Addison-Wesley, Massachusetts.

Hyland, M., Millard, J. and Parker, S. (1988) How hospital ward members treat learner nurses: an investigation of learners' perceptions in a British hospital. *Journal of Advanced Nursing*, **13**, 472–7.

Jacka, K. and Lewin, D. (1987) *The Clinical Learning of Student Nurses, NERU Report No. 6*, Kings College, London.

Jarvis, P. (1983) *Professional Education*, Croom Helm, London.

Jowett, S., Walton, I. and Payne, S. (1992) *Implementing Project 2000: an Interim Report*, National Foundation for Educational Research, Slough.

Lofland, J. and Lofland, L. (1984) *Analyzing Social Settings*, 2nd edn., Wadsworth, London.

McCaugherty, D. (1991) The theory-practice gap in nurse education: its causes and possible solutions. Findings from an action research study. *Journal of Advanced Nursing*, **16**, 1055–61.

Marriott, A. (1991) The support supervision and instruction of nurse learners in clinical areas: a literature review. *Nurse Education Today*, **11**, 261–9.

Marsh, C. (1982) *The Survey Method: the Contribution of Surveys to Sociological Explanation*, George Allen & Unwin, London.

Merriam, S. (1983) Mentors and proteges: A critical review of the literature. *Adult Education Quarterly*, **33**, 161–73.

Moser, C. and Stuart, A. (1953) An experimental study of quota sampling. *Journal of the Royal Statistical Society A*, **116**, 349–405.

Ogier, M. (1982) *An Ideal Sister?* Royal College of Nursing, London.

Orton, H., Prowse, J. and Millen, C. (1993) *Charting the Way to Excellence*, Health Research Centre, Sheffield Hallam University, Sheffield.

Pembrey, S. (1980) *The Ward Sister; Key to Nursing*, Royal College of Nursing, London.

Polgar, S. and Thomas, S. (1988) *Introduction to Research in the Health Sciences*, Churchill Livingstone, Edinburgh.

Reid, N. (1985) *Wards in Chancery?* Research Series, Royal College of Nursing, London.

Ryan, D. (1989) *Project 1999: the Support Hierarchy as the Management Contribution to Project 2000, Evaluation Project Discussion Paper No 4*, Department of Nursing Studies, University of Edinburgh, Edinburgh.

United Kingdom Central Council (1986) *Project 2000: A New Preparation for Practice*, United Kingdom Central Council for Nursing, Midwifery and Health Visiting, London.

While, A. (1991) The problem of clinical evaluation: a review. *Nurse Education Today*, **11**, 448–53.

White, E., Riley, E., Davies, S. and Twinn, S. (1994) *A Detailed Study of the Relationships Between Teaching, Support, Supervision and Role Modelling for Students in Clinical Areas, within the Context of Project 2000 Courses*. English National Board, London.

Yin, R. (1981) The case study crisis: some answers. *Administrative Science Quarterly*, **26**, 58–65.

Yin, R. (1984) *Case Study Research; Designs and Methods*, Sage Publications, London.

CHAPTER SEVEN

Stress and the community psychiatric nurse

Jerome Carson, Heather Bartlett,
Leonard Fagin, Daniel Brown and John Leary

INTRODUCTION

Concerns about stress in health care professionals have been highlighted in a number of research studies conducted in the 1980s (see Payne and Firth-Cozens, 1987, for a comprehensive review). More recently, the 'mental health of the NHS workforce' has been identified as one of five key priority areas in the Department of Health's research and development strategy. To date the bulk of the stress research literature has focused on either general nurses (Gray-Toft and Anderson, 1981), or on junior hospital doctors (Firth-Cozens, 1987). In turn, most of the nursing research has either concentrated on stressors specific to particular branches of nursing (Goodwin, 1983; Ehrenfeld and Cheifetz, 1990) or has concurrently compared several branches of nursing to identify which is the most stressful (Power and Sharp, 1988; Hipwell, Tyler and Wilson 1989; Foxall *et al.*, 1990). Other studies have tried to compare stress between different professional groups, and already the first professional stress league table has appeared in the literature (Rees and Smith, 1991). This burgeoning stress literature has not been confined to nursing alone. There are now published reports of stress in occupational therapists (Sweeney, Nichols and Kline, 1991), in social workers (Gibson, McGrath and Reid, 1989; Jones *et al.*, 1991; Bennett, Evans and Tattersall, 1993) and in clinical psychologists (Cushway, 1992). Psychiatrists would seem to be the only mental health professionals in this country to have avoided the close scrutiny of stress researchers. Margison (1987), however, provides some useful pointers for stress in psychiatrists.

The issue of stress in psychiatric nurses is not one that has been adequately addressed to date. In a review (Jones, 1987), only six studies could be identified worldwide that looked specifically at psychiatric nurses. Jones *et al.* (1987) described an investigation conducted into stress in psychiatric nursing, but this centred on the staff of one special hospital only. To our knowledge there have been no comparable studies of CPNs, with the exception of Handy's research (Handy, 1990). In her PhD thesis, Handy used qualitative methods to study stress from a sociopolitical perspective. CPNs, however, only formed a small part of Handy's study.

We begin the present account with a description of our initial pilot study, conducted in 1988.

THE PILOT STUDY

As is so often the case in research, our decision to start investigating the issue of stress and coping in CPNs occurred partly by chance. At the time Heather Bartlett was undertaking her specialist Registered Mental Nurse placement in the psychology department at Claybury Hospital. As part of his contribution to her placement experience, Jerome Carson suggested she do some research under his supervision and offered the topic of stress and coping in clinical psychologists. Heather suggested in return that she would be more interested in examining stress and coping among CPNs (possibly anticipating her future career choice!). A request for information to one of the district's senior nurses produced a surprisingly negative response, which paradoxically proved to be just the impetus needed to set up the pilot study. The aims of this study were firstly to try and develop a specific CPN stress questionnaire. We speculated that some of the stressors faced by CPNs would be different from ward-based colleagues. Our second aim was to identify what these stressors were. Thirdly, we wished to look at the type and amount of stress across four CPN departments. Finally we wanted to feed back the information from the study to all the districts who participated.

Our first task was to develop a specific measure of CPN stress. To do this we generated a large pool of potential items. These were taken from 16 individual interviews that Heather conducted with different grades of CPN in the four survey districts. Respondents were simply asked 'What stresses you in your job as a CPN?' All their answers were recorded. The resulting pool of items was eventually reduced to 66. Each item was scored on a five-point scale, where 0 = 'This causes me no stress', to 4 = 'This causes me extreme stress'. Subsequent work by our team, looking at the sensitivity of each item and at item total correlations, has further reduced the questionnaire to its present format of 48 items. A paper on the psychometric properties of the new scale will be available shortly (Brown *et al.*, 1994a).

The CPN Stress Questionnaire thus developed was then administered, along with the Maslach Burnout Inventory (Maslach and Jackson, 1986) and the General Health Questionnaire GHQ-28 (Goldberg and Williams, 1988), to 61 CPNs in four districts. Response rates averaged over 90%, as we gave the questionnaires to staff via departmental meetings. We chose to use the Maslach Burnout Inventory and General Health Questionnaire as they are both well-standardized scales that have been used in research studies throughout the world. The Maslach Burnout Inventory comprises three subscales: emotional exhaustion, depersonalization and personal accomplishment. The General Health Questionnaire, GHQ-28, has four subscales covering somatic symptoms, anxiety and insomnia, social role functioning and severe depression. In non-clinical samples subscale scores are often low, so the most important score is the Total GHQ Score. Of interest also is the number of subjects that score as 'cases', that is subjects scoring 5 or more on the scale. Both the Maslach and the GHQ-28 have the advantage of being short, easy to score and quick to administer.

On the CPN Stress Questionnaire the most stressful items were as follows.

1. Not having facilities in the community that I can refer my clients on to.
2. Working with clients with a history of violence.
3. Having too many interruptions in the office.
4. Visiting unpredictable clients.
5. Knowing there are long waiting lists before my clients can get access to services.
6. Dealing with suicidal clients on my own.
7. Visiting unsafe areas.
8. Not being informed of treatment changes affecting my client.
9. Communication problems with other professionals.
10. Having to work with resistive couples or families.
11. Covering for colleagues on sick leave or holiday.

The maximum possible score on the Questionnaire was 264, but individual scores ranged from 7 to 187, with an average of 99.03. There were no significant differences in scores across the four departments. Interestingly, in the department which had the lowest score more than half the CPNs scored more than the average of 99, showing that one or two low scorers had artificially pulled the departmental average down.

The average Total GHQ Score was 3.02, with 23% of the sample scoring five or above, the so-called 'caseness' level. One in five CPNs could be said to be psychologically distressed at the time they completed the Questionnaire. On the Maslach Burnout Inventory emotional exhaustion subscale, 24% had high scores. The average score was 19.07, slightly higher than the figures obtained by Firth and his colleagues (1987). On the depersonalization subscale (which measures empathic relationship with patients) the majority of CPNs, 81%, scored in the low category; average score was 4.15, well below the 6.1

average reported by Firth. Scores were more evenly distributed on the personal accomplishment subscale, though our average, 32.48, was lower and therefore worse than the 36.5 reported by Firth. Again here there were no significant differences between the four districts.

It would be fair to say that we were surprised by some of our findings. For instance that 'having too many interruptions in the office' was seen as the third most stressful event seemed to contradict the enthusiasm of planners to put all CPNs into one large open-plan office. Clinical concerns, such as dealing with violent and suicidal clients, were predictably high on the list, and serve to emphasize the different approach required from staff in community settings (Butterworth and Skidmore, 1981). The study found that one in five CPNs was psychologically distressed and four out of 10 had low personal accomplishment scores, not seeing themselves as very effective or achieving in their work. At the time (Carson, Bartlett and Croucher, 1991), we suggested that the rapid pace of changes in the Health Service made the monitoring of staff stress levels even more urgent. With hindsight, this seems a prophetic statement.

STRESS AND ORGANIZATIONAL CHANGE – SCHAFER'S STUDY

Tim Schafer was one of the first researchers to use our own methodology in a study of organizational change in West Essex (Schafer, 1992). We had surveyed the West Essex CPNs some months before this district changed the management structure, splitting the department up into three functional units. The CPNs had previously been one cohesive unit with their own senior nurse manager. Schafer studied Korner returns for the quarter preceding the organizational change, and for a quarter commencing 6 months after the changes had taken place. Total referrals increased from 211 to 396, an 88% rise. There was also a 41% increase in the number of patient visits. At the same time there were increases in measured stress among CPNs. The mean GHQ-28 score rose from 3.21 to 5.00, with the Maslach emotional exhaustion scale rising from 19 to 23.56. The depersonalization score rose also from 4.07 to 5.31. The personal accomplishment score, in contrast, had also risen slightly. So while CPNs were more stressed after the change, they perceived themselves to be more effective in their role.

Perhaps the most interesting findings from Schafer's study concerned the CPN Stress Questionnaire. Average scores here had risen by almost 10 points from 91.93 to 101.2. Schafer noted a number of changes in the items that were causing CPNs to feel stressed. Two major factors that had changed after the managerial reorganizations were that CPNs reported supervision issues to be a significant concern, along with complaints about the managerial changes themselves. Schafer concluded that the CPN Stress Questionnaire was a sensitive and discriminating assessment tool and that it should be used periodically within CPN departments to help monitor stress among staff.

ADDING A QUALITATIVE DIMENSION – THE Q-SORT STUDY

One of the biggest gaps in our first study was a lack of information on CPNs' coping strategies. To find out how CPNs' coped with work stress, Tim Gallagher, a psychology student, interviewed 21 CPNs on our behalf, using a semi-structured interview. There were 13 specific questions, e.g. 'What is the best way of handling stress at work from your viewpoint?' (Question 1); 'What makes your own working life easier?' (Question 3). The results of these interviews are partially reported in a *Nursing Times* paper (Carson *et al.*, 1993). We used this material to generate a pack of 61 Q-statements for a Coping Q-Sort. A second Q-Sort pack was derived from our CPN Stress Questionnaire, with 60 stress statements. The Coping Q-Sort and the Stress Q-Sort were then administered to 44 CPNs in four health districts. Both packs of Q-Sort statements were individually printed on to white cards. Packs were shuffled and given to respondents who were asked to place each statement relative to the others on to a large normal distribution template with 'strongly agree' at one pole, and 'strongly disagree' at the other. Half of the subjects were given the Coping Q-Sort first, and the other half the Stress Q-Sort. This is in line with established Q-Sort methodology (Stephenson, 1936). For each Q-Sort the three statements most strongly disagreed with were given a rank of 1, the four statements next agreed with a value of 2 and so on. The nine neutral statements received a value of 6, and the three most agreed with a value of 11. These data were compiled and subjected to factor analysis, in common with other similar studies (Kitzinger and Rogers, 1985). This resulted in nine factors for the stress array and 12 for the coping array. Both factors were rotated to simple structure (varimax criterion). Gallagher (1992) gave idiosyncratic labels to some of the factors emerging. For instance he labelled two of the stress discourses as: 'There's only one of me and I don't like suicidal clients' (Factor 3) and 'Don't interrupt me I need colleagues' (Factor 9). Some of the labels he gave the coping discourses were as follows: 'The right person, supported, copes' (Factor 5) and 'Don't try, the boss doesn't listen' (Factor 9). The results of the Stress Q-Sort have validated constructs used in our CPN Stress Questionnaire. Issues such as personal safety, violent patients and interruptions in the office were chosen for the extremes of the stress discourses.

The study did however demonstrate that there was a greater consensus on what is stressful (nine separate viewpoints), than on how to cope with it (12 viewpoints). It has also found stress and coping to be a complex web of interdependent perceptions and attributions. A further paper on this work will be available shortly.

THE CLAYBURY CPN STRESS STUDY

Towards the end of 1992, we received a grant from the North East Thames Regional Health Authority's Local Organized Research Scheme (LORS) to conduct a major investigation of stress and coping in CPNs. The main objectives of the study were:

1. to examine the variety, frequency and severity of stressors among CPNs in the North East Thames Region;
2. to examine the coping strategies used by CPNs to reduce their levels of occupational stress;
3. to compare CPNs with hospital-based psychiatric nurses;
4. to provide feedback on the study's findings to all individuals and districts who have participated in the study;
5. to provide recommendations to CPNs and their managers on work stressors and effective coping strategies;
6. to disseminate the findings of the study to a wider audience.

There were two major parts to the research, a quantitative element and a qualitative component. For the quantitative part a range of questionnaires were given to all CPNs within the North East Thames Region. This involved survey-ing 15 districts, with only one refusing to participate. The measures we used were:

1. a demographic questionnaire (a measure specially developed by us, and available from the first author);
2. the CPN Stress Questionnaire (Revised) (Brown *et al.*, 1994a);
3. the Maslach Burnout Inventory (Maslach and Jackson, 1986);
4. the General Health Questionnaire (GHQ-28) (Goldberg and Williams, 1988);
5. the Modified Rosenberg Self-Esteem Scale (Wycherley, 1987);
6. the Minnesota Job Satisfaction Scale (Koelbel, Fuller and Misener, 1991);
7. the Coping Skills measure from Cooper's Occupational Stress Indicator (Cooper, Sloan and Williams, 1988).

We were able to administer this batch of questionnaires to 250 CPNs, each of whom received an individualized feedback form on their own results. Additionally each department received a general report and a presentation of its own findings. Feedback on a regional basis took place at a conference held at Claybury Hospital on 19 November 1993. The same questionnaires, with the exception of our CPN measure, were given to 323 ward-based psychiatric nurses drawn from five psychiatric hospitals and two general hospital psychiatric units. Initial findings from the quantitative research have been reported (Brown *et al.*, 1994b).

The qualitative element of the study involved randomly allocating CPN departments for individual interviews or group discussions. Within each district, volunteers were sought to participate in this second phase of the research. This work is still ongoing; results from the qualitative work will be reported in a new book which will give much more detail on the study and its findings (Carson, Fagin and Ritter, 1994).

Again, the CPN Stress Questionnaire (Revised) has provided us with some of the most intriguing findings. The top 10 stressors are now the following.

1. Not having facilities in the community that you can refer clients on to.
2. Knowing there are likely to be long waiting lists before clients can get access to services.
3. Having to deal with suicidal clients on your own.
4. Not having enough time for study or personal improvement.
5. Trying to keep up a good quality of care in your work.
6. Having too many interruptions when trying to work in the office.
7. Having to visit unsafe areas.
8. Feeling there is not enough hospital back-up.
9. Having to work with clients with a known history of violence.
10. Having to cope with changes at your workbase.

Surprisingly, six out of the 10 items are identical to the main stressors identified in our pilot study. These were items 1,2,3,6,7 and 9. If we look at the top third scorers on the CPN Stress Questionnaire (Revised), and we compare them with the bottom third, i.e. the least stressed CPNs, a number of interesting and statistically significant differences emerge. The mean GHQ score for our low-stress group was 2.5, but for the high stress group it was 7.7. Maslach emotional exhaustion scores for the low-stress group averaged 14.5 and for the high stress group 28.8. CPNs scoring low on our CPN Stress Questionnaire took on average 4.8 days off sick in the last year. For the high-stress group the number of sickness days was 11.1.

On the General Health Questionnaire, the average for CPNs is now 4.80 (SD = 5.8), which is much higher than the 3.02 reported in our pilot study. CPNs scored significantly higher than ward staff, whose average score was 3.4 (SD = 4.4). In terms of 'caseness', 41% of CPNs scored five or above, in comparison with 28% of the ward staff. The percentage of CPN cases is virtually double that in our pilot study. The average scores on Maslach's Burnout Inventory were higher on this occasion on both emotional exhaustion and depersonalization. CPNs would seem to be more burned out now than before.

IMPLICATIONS OF THE STRESS RESEARCH

Our own research on CPNs joins a wide body of research on other health care professionals which highlights the pressures facing workers. Such research leads inexorably to the question: what can be done to reduce the stress of CPNs?

Stress-reducing interventions can be applied at a variety of levels. Firstly, individual CPNs who have problems coping might be offered individual stress management courses. Scondly, a group of CPNs within a district service might be offered a group-based approach tailored to their local circumstances.

This might cover broader issues such as how to obtain more resources from their organization. Thirdly, health providers might be encouraged to offer stress reduction packges for all staff, of which CPNs constitute only a small part. Here the organization would attempt to meet its responsibilities in caring for the carers. Fourthly, and perhaps most contentiously, it might be helpful to monitor the effects of wider-scale service changes on CPNs. For instance, how has the change to GP fundholding affected stress levels in CPNs? How much additional stress has the extra bureaucracy that this entails caused CPNs involved with such schemes? Even stating the options in this simplistic way reveals the paucity of intervention research in this field.

One approach developed recently is social support group therapy (Carson, 1994). This approach derives from a number of different research sources, looking at the beneficial effects of belonging to a group. Peer support is probably the single most important coping strategy reported by staff in most research studies of professional groups. Social support group therapy aims to help staff maximize their psychological functioning through the development of effective personal support systems. The approach has recently been piloted on nursing staff in the Bethlem and Maudsley Special Health Authority and is currently being compared against cognitive therapy in a large field trial being conducted by Judy Proudfoot at the Institute of Psychiatry. Intuitively, it appears likely that the most effective approach to stress management in CPNs requires tackling it at different levels and not just social support. Time management (Fontana, 1993), for example, is just one of a series of skills that CPNs will require to function effectively in the community. Comprehensive approaches also need to take account of the specific occupational stressors noted by our own research. 'Having too many interruptions while trying to work in the office' was rated as the sixth most stressful event for CPNs. While a number of practical solutions to this problem can be identified, such as having a rota to answer the phone or partitioning noisy offices, the problem would be solved if CPNs had their own offices! This would indeed be a luxury for many CPNs. Indeed during the group discussions that were conducted as part of the qualitative phase of our research, one CPN told how three community occupational therapists arrived one day and asked to use her desk. They had been told that the CPN only used the desk for part of the day! Safety issues also featured prominently in CPNs' stress list. 'Having to visit unsafe areas' often presented more anxieties for the CPN than working with the clients themselves. Joint visits have to be considered in this situation, although in the present cost-conscious economic climate this might not always be feasible. The practical concerns arising from our research suggest that comprehensive stress management approaches need to address these wider issues as well. We now await the first attempts to deliver such packages to CPNs in the field.

CONCLUSIONS

We began this chapter by describing our first pilot study on stress among CPNs, conducted in 1988. We then talked about Schafer's extension of our work. We described the Q-Sort study, our next research project. Finally we gave a description of the Claybury CPN Stress Study and presented some preliminary data on this. In terms of future research there are a number of avenues worth exploring. There is a clear need for more longitudinal work, especially of temporal changes in stress levels as a function of different expectations and alterations in individuals' job characteristics. Cross-sectional studies obviously do not provide this detail as easily. There is also a need to develop stress management techniques that will help CPNs manage more effectively. Although techniques such as social skills have been shown not to be very effective with very disabled clients, they may prove more helpful if offered to groups of staff. Finally there is a need to replicate our own findings elsewhere.

It might be the case that the North East Thames Region is not typical of other parts of the country. While nurses nationally have been subjected to 'regrading', and many are now experiencing 'downgrading', we would urge managers to proceed cautiously in managing change, as nursing is not only one of the key health service professions, it is also a stressful one.

ACKNOWLEDGEMENTS

We are indebted to a large number of colleagues for their guidance and assistance in developing our research ideas. We wish to thank especially Professors Wakeling, Butterworth, Gournay, Yule and Cooper, Drs Beardsell, Sanderson, Stainton-Rogers, Boyle and Brooker and also Ed White, Christine Hancock, Malcolm Scott and Sue Ritter. Most especially we are grateful to all the community psychiatric nurses and their managers who have been the participants in our research. We sincerely hope that their hard effort has been rewarded by our research endeavours. Finally we acknowledge the secretarial back-up of Fenella Cardwell and Norma Matthews.

REFERENCES

Bennett, P., Evans, R. and Tattersall, A. (1993) Stress and coping in social workers: a preliminary investigation. *British Journal of Social Work*, **23**, 31–44.

Brown, D., Carson, J., Fagin, L. *et al*. (1994a) Evaluating the mental health of mental health nursing staff – a comparison of hospital and community based psychiatric nurses. *Nursing Times*, submitted for publication.

Brown, D., Leary, J., Bartlett, H. *et al.* (1994b) Stress in community psychiatric nurses: the development of a measure. *British Journal of Clinical Psychology*, submitted for publication.

Butterworth, A. and Skidmore, D. (1981) *Caring for the Mentally Ill in the Community*, Croom Helm, Beckenham.

Carson, J. (1994) Social support group therapy – treatment manual. Unpublished manuscript available from the first author.

Carson, J., Bartlett, H. and Croucher, P. (1991) Stress in community psychiatric nurses: a preliminary investigation. *Community Psychiatric Nursing Journal*, 2, 8–13.

Carson, J., Bartlett, H., Leary, J. *et al.* (1993) Stress and the CPN. *Nursing Times*, 89, 38–40.

Carson, J., Fagin, L. and Ritter, S. (1994) *Stress and Coping in Mental Health*, Chapman & Hall, London.

Cooper, C., Sloan, S. and Williams, S. (1988) *Occupational Stress Indicator*, NFER-Nelson, Windsor.

Cushway, C. (1992) Stress in clinical psychology trainees. *British Journal of Clinical Psychology*, 31, 169–79.

Ehrenfeld, M. and Cheifetz, F. (1990) Cardiac nurses coping with stress. *Journal of Advanced Nursing*, 15, 1002–8.

Firth, H., McKeown, P., McIntee, J. and Britton, P. (1987) Burn out personality and support in long stay nursing. *Nursing Times*, 83, 55–7.

Firth-Cozens, J. (1987) Emotional distress in junior house officers. *British Medical Journal*, 195, 522–36.

Fontana, D. (1993) *Managing Time*, British Psychological Society, Leicester.

Foxall, M., Zimmerman, L., Standley, R. and Bene, B. (1990) A comparison of frequency and sources of nursing job related stress perceived by intensive care, hospice and medical surgical nurses. *Journal of Advanced Nursing*, 15, 577–84.

Gallagher, T. (1992) A Q-methodological study of stress and coping mechanisms in the community psychiatric nurse. University of East London. BSc Thesis.

Gibson, F., McGrath, A. and Reid, N. (1989) Occupational stress in social work. *British Journal of Social Work*, 19, 1–16.

Goldberg, D. and Williams, P. (1988) *A User's Guide to the General Health Questionnaire*, NFER-Nelson, Windsor.

Goodwin, S. (1983) The stresses of health visiting. *Health Visitor*, 56, 20–1.

Gray-Toft, P. and Anderson, J. (1981) Stress amongst hospital nursing staff: its causes and effects. *Social Science and Medicine*, 15, 639–47.

Handy, J. (1990) *Occupational Stress in a Caring Profession*, Gower, Aldershot.

Hipwell, A., Tyler, P. and Wilson, C. (1989) Sources of stress and dissatisfaction among nurses in four hospital environments. *British Journal of Medical Psychology*, 62, 71–9.

Jones, J.G. (1987) Stress in psychiatric nursing, in *Stress in Health Professionals*, (eds R. Payne and J. Firth-Cozens), John Wiley, Chichester.

Jones, J.G., Janman, K., Payne, R. and Rick, J. (1987) Some determinants of stress in psychiatric nurses. *International Journal of Nursing Studies*, 28, 29–45.

Kitzinger, C. and Rogers, R. (1985) A Q-methodological study of lesbian identity. *European Journal of Social Psychology*, 15, 167–87.

Koelbel, P., Fuller, F. and Misener, T. (1991) Job satisfaction of nurse practitioners: an analysis using Herzberg's theory. *Nurse Practitioner*, **16**, 43–56.

Margison, F. (1987) Stress in psychiatrists, in *Stress in Health Professionals*, (eds R. Payne and J. Firth-Cozens), John Wiley, Chichester.

Maslach, C. and Jackson, S. (1986) *Maslach Burnout Inventory*, Consulting Psychologists Press, California.

Payne, R. and Firth-Cozens, J. (eds) (1987) *Stress in Health Professionals*, John Wiley, Chichester.

Power, K. and Sharp, G. (1988) A comparison of sources of nursing stress and job satisfaction among mental handicap and hospice nursing staff. *Journal of Advanced Nursing*, **13**, 726–32.

Rees, D. and Smith, S. (1991) Work stress in occupational therapists asssessed by the occupational stress indicator. *British Journal of Occupational Therapy*, **54**, 289–94.

Schafer, T. (1992) CPN stress and organisational change: a study. *Community Psychiatric Nursing Journal*, **1**, 16–24.

Stephenson, W. (1936) A new application of correlations to averages. *British Journal of Educational Psychology*, **6**, 43–57.

Sweeney, G., Nichols, K. and Kline, P. (1991) Factors contributing to work related stress in occupational therapists. *British Journal of Occupational Therapy*, **54**, 284–8.

Wycherley, B. (1987) *The Living Skills Pack*. South East Thames Regional Health Authority, Bexhill.

CHAPTER EIGHT

Targeting services for seriously mentally ill people: implications for community psychiatric nurses

Julie Repper and Rachel Perkins

OVERVIEW OF POLICY AND RESEARCH FINDINGS

The development of local community-based care has been explicit mental health policy for almost three decades (DHSS, 1975; DoH, 1990a) and it has been recognized that the real challenge for community services, and the measure of their success, is the extent to which they meet the needs of people with severe and long-term mental illness (DHSS, 1981; Reed, 1991). Indeed, all recent mental health policy legislation has explicitly prioritized this client group (DoH 1989a, b, 1990b, c, 1991, 1992). Despite these policy intentions, there is considerable evidence that specific targeting of these most disabled clients has not occurred and that community services have failed to meet the needs of, and engage, many who require their input.

Most of those people who experience serious long-term mental health problems are in the care of generic 'patch' or community mental health teams who have a responsibility for serving all those with mental health problems in a given area (Jenkins, 1989). Nurses working in such teams spend most of their time with clients who experience acute and neurotic illnesses (Wooff and Goldberg, 1988). A recent study revealed that in 1989 a quarter of all CPNs in England had not a single client with a diagnosis of schizophrenia on their caseloads (White, 1993), and Brooker (1990) showed that projects undertaken by trainee CPNs rarely focused on people with severe mental llness. This generic team model of service provision has therefore, apparently, failed to target the most disabled groups in the manner that policy has dictated. This targeting failure has led some to argue that specialist rehabilitation and continuing care teams are necessary if the needs of severely mentally ill people are to be met (Olfsen, 1990; Meltzer *et al.*, 1991). However, even within such specialist teams appropriate targeting is not guaranteed; Sayce, Craig and Boardman (1991) reported that within services explicitly dedicated to people with long-term mental illness there is a tendency to move 'up market' towards client groups who are more likely to 'get better'.

Although studies of resettlement projects for long-stay hospital patients have reported some success (Jones, Robinson and Golightly, 1986; Knapp *et al.*, 1990; Milner, 1991), and research has demonstrated that care in the community can be effective for severely disabled people who have never been chronically institutionalized (Stein and Test, 1980; Hoult and Reynolds, 1983; Dean and Gadd, 1990), there is worrying evidence that a considerable number of seriously mentally ill people remain in hospital because community support services are inadequate to their needs (O'Driscoll, Marshall and Reed, 1990; Holloway *et al.*, 1988).

Many of those who do live in the community fail to receive the care they need and have been found to: become extremely socially isolated (Beels *et al.*, 1984); spend a great deal of their time doing very little (Warden, Walsh and Becker, 1990); have undiagnosed and untreated physical health problems (Koran *et al.*, 1989; Wells *et al.*, 1989); be at risk of physical violence and exploitation (Bachrach, 1984); fall foul of the criminal justice system (Coid, 1988); become homeless (Timms and Fry, 1989; Weller, 1989); and live in impoverished conditions (Johnstone *et al.*, 1984).

There is considerable evidence that, among severely mentally ill 'new long-term' clients (Shepherd, 1984) who have never been chronically institutionalized, there are people who frequently drop out of community services or underuse them (Prevost, 1989; Bachrach, 1982; Perkins and Rowland, 1986; Belcher, 1988; Reed, 1991). Bender and Pilling (1985), for example, found that people with long-term mental illness were least likely to engage in a mental health day centre, and Meltzer *et al.* (1991) reported very low levels of engagement in day care and supported accommodation amongst profoundly disabled people with a diagnosis of schizophrenia with active symptomatology. Hirsch *et al.* (1992, p. 4) described

> a group of patients who are hard to sustain in a meaningful clinical alliance with psychiatric services. . . . These patients do not engage in treatment, are often not at home when the doctors, nurses or social workers visit and may abuse alcohol, lack insight or withdraw themselves from treatment. They sometimes end up with no home of their own.

Clearly the acceptability and accessibility of services to the clients for whom they are designed is of central importance.

In addition to underengagement – reflecting the acceptability of the service to the client – there is also the issue of the acceptability of the client to the service. Some severely disabled people are specifically denied access to community care services. Several authors have suggested that clients may be appropriately referred for community care services, but rejected by those services because they are deemed unamenable to treatment by virtue of a diagnosis of personality disorder, forensic history, potential violence and/or learning disabilities (Showalter, 1987; Hirsch *et al.*, 1992). Similarly Bachrach (1982) suggests that patients who are deemed to be 'difficult' and who engender negative feelings in staff are often rejected or even actively 'blacklisted' by community services.

THE CLIENTS: UNDERSTANDING THEIR PROBLEMS AND NEEDS

People with serious mental health problems are a diverse group comprising people with a huge range of backgrounds, needs, circumstances and diagnoses. Some old long-stay patients have lived in hospital for many years and grown old there but, in the present era of deinstitutionalization, it is more typical for severely mentally ill people to be maintained in the community for most of the time with only brief stays in hospital at times of crisis. There are, of course, a small group of 'new long-stay patients' whom community services have failed to maintain in community living, and the size of this group clearly depends upon the quality and extent of community care provided. If institutionalization is to become a thing of the past then the community care needs of those more disabled new long-term and new long-stay clients are paramount.

Serious ongoing mental health problems not infrequently render a person 'socially disabled' – unable to perform socially to the standards expected by themselves, those important to them or society in general (Wing and Morris, 1981). Such social disability arises as a consequence of four factors: the person's symptoms (both positive and negative); the way in which they cope with and adapt to the experience of mental illness; the personal, social and material resources available to them to facilitate such adaptation; and the numerous social disadvantages, such as poverty, stigma, bars to employment, that the experience of mental illness in our society brings (Wing and Morris, 1981; Shepherd, 1984).

For people who are socially disabled as a consequence of ongoing mental health problems the traditional 'treatment/cure' approach focused on problem removal is of limited utility. As with any ongoing disability, whether it be physical or psychiatric, interventions need to be directed towards optimizing and maintaining functioning (Shepherd, 1984), enhancing quality of life (Lehman, Ward and Linn, 1982; Thapa and Rowland, 1989) and relationships (Perkins and Dilks, 1992), and ensuring that the person has access to social activities and facilities (Shepherd, 1984) so that they can take their rightful place as respected citizens of our communities. This means that a multi-faceted psychosocial approach is required both to understand the difficulties experienced and to ameliorate distress and disability. Given the nature of social disability a narrow, symptom-oriented, biological approach is insufficient and grossly inappropriate.

The extent of a person's disability depends not only upon characteristics, skills and problems of the individual, but also upon the characteristics of the environment in which they are required to function. In the same way as physical disability, social disability can only be defined in relation to the demands and expectations that society imposes. Therefore a major component of providing effective services for severely socially disabled people revolves around understanding the social circumstances in which they are required to function, the enabling or disabling impact of these and the ways in which supports can be provided and the social environment adapted to minimize disability.

THE STUDIES

In order to contribute to a better understanding of the needs of this client group and the ways in which services might more appropriately be targeted to meet these needs, two studies will be reported in this chapter. The first will offer an overview of a population of long-term mental health service users from an inner London borough in terms of their demographic and psychiatric characteristics and the services that they use. By examining a district's entire population of long-term service users this study gives an indication of the characteristics of long-term clients that a CPN working in a generic catchment area team might expect to encounter. The second will describe the population of severely socially disabled people referred to a specialist rehabilitation and community care service in Nottingham, including the characteristics of those who were not accepted into care or themselves found the services unacceptable and refused input. The more in-depth information about the subgroup of long-term service users who are referred to a specialist rehabilitation team has implications for CPNs working as keyworkers or case managers in such more specialist settings.

LONG-TERM MENTAL HEALTH SERVICE USERS IN AN INNER LONDON BOROUGH

Wandsworth is a multiracial, relatively deprived inner London borough. The mental health services provided to the population of the area (population 191 250) by the district Community and Specialist Mental Health Services had as their core a series of patch-based multidisciplinary community mental health teams (CMHTs). There was also a specialist rehabilitation and long-term care team providing care for those who were the most disabled by their serious and persistent mental health problems, a service for elderly people and a series of highly specialized regional and supraregional services including a mother and baby unit and behaviour therapy, eating disorders, developmental disorders, deaf and drug misuse services. CPNs were attached to and had a key role within all of the CMHTs and more specialist services and keyworker and multidisciplinary care planning systems were in operation.

A network of supported and sheltered accommodation, work and day care/drop-in services was provided by health and social services and the voluntary sector in the area. For those most severely disabled by their mental health problems, there were 'hospital hostels' – houses both on and off the hospital site staffed and run by the rehabilitation team – and a network of houses owned by housing associations where residents had secured tenancies and were provided with support by rehabilitation team members. This support ranged from 24-hour on-site cover to peripatetic input 7 days per week.

Since 1990 an annually updated 'long-term care case register' has provided information on the demographic, psychiatric, functioning and service usage characteristics of all long-term mental health service users in the area. The data reported here were collected as part of the 1993 update of this case register.

Method

Subject. Data were collected on all those people who were in contact with Pathfinder community and specialist services for Wandsworth clients (excluding drug misuse, forensic and psychotherapy service clients) on 1 April 1993, who were aged between 16 and 75 years and who had their first contact with adult mental health services at least 2 years previously (on or before 1 April 1991). It was decided not simply to include those who had been in continuous contact with mental health services because this would exclude those people with long-term problems who move into and out of service care, especially that group of younger, severely disabled 'revolving door' clients that all mental health services have most difficulties in engaging (Meltzer *et al.*, 1991).

Data collection and procedure. On a specially designed form, data were collected for all long-term clients concerning demographic characteristics (age, sex, race, accommodation, occupation, etc.), service usage (patient status, professionals in contact, day time facilities used, etc.), and psychiatric/ functioning variables (diagnosis, number of hospitalizations, duration of contact with services, role functioning, etc.). The clients on whom data were collected were identified from team and service records and their keyworkers then provided with the necessary information. All keyworkers were told that the information they provided should be correct as at 1 April 1993.

Table 8.1 Characteristics of long-term mental health service users in the London Borough of Wandsworth, 1993 (population 191 250)

Total number of long-term mental health service users	1071 (560/100 000 population)
CMHTs	883(55.4% of CMHT clients)
Specialist rehabilitation team	97(9.0%)
Other specialist teams	91(8.5%)
Female (%)	55.6
Mean age (SD)	45.0 years (13.8)
Single, divorced, widowed or separated (%)	73.0
Race/ethnicity (%)	
UK/Irish	67.0
African Caribbean	15.6
Asian	8.1
Mean no. of years since first contact with psychiatric services (SD)	15.3(10.5)
No. of admissions (%)	
None	18
One	16
Two to five	41
Six or more	25
Primary diagnosis (%)	
Schizophrenia	44
Depression	17
Manic-depressive illness	15
Anxiety-based problems	8
Schizo-affective disorder	5
Personality disorder	4
Drug/alcohol abuse	4
Usual accommodation (%)	
Inpatient	
1990	10
1993	4

(63% of inpatients live in 'hospital hostels' – hospital-owned and -staffed houses on or off the hospital site)

Supported accommodation in community	
1990	12
1993	16
Independent accommodation in community	
1990	77
1993	80

Table 8.1 *contd*

Living arrangements (%)	
Alone	51
With spouse/cohabitee	28
Lone adult with children	7
With parents	11
Occupational status (%)	
In open employment	16
In sheltered work	8
Unemployed	54
Retired	12
Some form of structured daytime activity (%)	52.1
Multidisciplinary input (%)	
At least two professions in contact	53
At least three professions in contact	23
Professions in contact (%)	
Psychiatrist	78
CPN	40
Social worker	25
Occupational therapist	18
Psychologist	11
No. of new long-term clients entering the care of services in the year 1992/1993 (pop. 191 250)	46
No. of long-term clients entering the care of services in the year 1992/1993	206
No. of long-term clients leaving the care of services	
1991	168 (51% dropped out)
1992	211 (33% dropped out)
1993	300 (21% dropped out)
Role disturbance (%)	
Unable to get work/in imminent danger of being sacked	64.0
Unable to carry out usual family roles	41.7
Isolated and lacking social support	43.6
At risk of losing current accommodation	4.4
Unable to manage finances without help	20.5
Causing disturbances in the community	9.5
	(55% show marked disturbance in at least two of the above areas; 34% in at least three)

Results

Table 8.1 shows that on 1 April 1993 there were 1071 long-term service users in the care of the mental health services for Wandsworth: 560 per 100 000 of population. With a mean age of 45 years, most had experienced mental health problems for many years – an average of over 15 years had elapsed since their first contact with psychiatric services. They were predominantly single, living alone, few (16%) had jobs in open employment and only slightly over half had any form of structured daytime activity (52.1%). The vast majority had been admitted to psychiatric hospital at least once (82%) and most (66%) had experienced multiple admissions: one-quarter had been admitted at least six times.

It is sometimes assumed that all long-term service users have schizophrenia. This is not the case. Although the largest proportion of this population had a diagnosis of schizophrenia (44%), more than half did not: there were substantial numbers with a primary diagnosis of some form of affective disorder and 8% had anxiety-based problems of long standing. They did, however, show marked impairment of social role functioning. Over 60% were unable to work as a consequence of their mental health problems and substantial proportions experienced marked disturbance of functioning within their family and were socially isolated and lacking in social support. This indicates the need for vocational, family and social interventions, in addition to specific symptom management in work with this group.

It should also be noted that over one-fifth were unable to manage their finances unaided. This was a particularly critical problem in relation to a person's community tenure; difficulties with money are not infrequently associated with acute hospital admissions as demands for bills to be paid are not only stressful but may result in disconnection of electricity, gas, telephone or, at worst, eviction. That the majority were multiply, but not universally, disabled can be seen from the fact that some 55% had marked disturbance in role functioning in at least two of the areas considered, and over one-third had marked impairments in at least three.

Despite this level of social role disturbance, the majority (96%) lived in the community: some (16%) in supported/sheltered facilities but most (80%) in their own independent accommodation receiving outpatient, day and outreach support, the latter often provided by CPNs. Developments in community care for long-term clients can be seen in the reduction of long-term inpatients from 10% of the long-term population in 1990 to only 4% in 1993. Of the remaining long-term inpatients, the majority (3%) did not live in ward accommodation: most lived in staffed houses on and off the hospital site.

It is important to note that the specialist rehabilitation and continuing care team provided care for only a small (albeit particularly disabled) proportion of the population of long-term service users (9%). The majority (82.5%) were in the care of the patch CMHTs: long-term clients comprised 55% of the

CMHTs' caseload. This indicates that support for people with long-term mental health problems should not be a small, specialist, enterprise but a substantial and important part of the work of all generic mental health professionals. Although the majority (78%) were in regular contact with a psychiatrist, of the other professionals in the multidisciplinary team it was clearly CPNs who had a central and important role in the care of this group. Some 40% of long-term service users had regular CPN input – such clients comprised a substantial proportion of CPNs' caseloads, as indicated by the national picture referred to earlier.

It is a reflection of the heterogeneity of long-term clients' problems that many required the input and expertise of a variety of different professionals. Over half were in regular contact with staff from at least two professions and almost one-quarter had input from at least three. This means that multidisciplinary care planning and coordination is crucial. If a person is receiving input from different people then problems of duplication and omission all too easily occur; it is not uncommon for everyone to assume that someone else is dealing with a particular difficulty.

Although many long-term clients remain in continuous service contact for long periods of time, it is important to recognize that people do enter and leave service care as their needs change. In the year 1992/1993 300 long-term clients left service care and over 200 entered it, but only 46 of these were 'new' long-term clients for whom 2 years had only just elapsed since their first contact with mental health services. The remainder were people who had experienced problems for many years and who re-entered service care. Long-term mental health problems are notoriously variable: a person who requires a high level of care at one time may require little or none at another. While it is clearly important that services are responsive to the changing needs of those who remain in their care, it is also important that people can enter and leave services as their needs dictate; services must be readily accessible for those with long-term problems who require only intermittent service input.

Finally, the problem of 'drop-out' is evident from the figures presented in Table 8.1. Of the 300 long-term clients who left care in 1992/1993 over one-fifth dropped out or refused all the care they were deemed to need by service providers. Although moves to reduce the rate of drop-out by more effectively tailoring care to clients' needs (including discharging them when their needs dictated) had reduced the drop-out rate from 51% of those leaving support in 1990/1991 to 21% in 1992/1993, the ways in which care can be rendered acceptable to those who need it remain an issue for all professionals.

REFERRALS TO A SPECIALIST REHABILITATION AND COMMUNITY CARE SERVICE IN NOTTINGHAM

Nottingham district mental health services serve a population of 600 000 people, three-quarters of whom live in the relatively compact conurbation of Nottingham. Taken as a whole, the district is typical in broad sociodemo-graphic terms of cities of its size, but there exist a wide range of differences between inner city and rural areas.

Acute psychiatric services operated on a sectorized patch system of multidisciplinary clinical teams and there was a specialist Rehabilitation and Community Care Service (RCCS) that was designed to provide care for clients who were more disabled by long-term problems. Unlike the previous study, which looked at an entire population of long-term service users and the services they received, the purpose of this study was to focus on the work of this specialist rehabilitation team and in particular to consider the characteristics of those referred to this specialist team and the implications of these in more detail.

Within Nottingham there were a range of accommodation, work and day facilities provided by voluntary agencies, and social services and the RCCS itself provided a comprehensive range of residential, work, day, drop-in and outreach services for approximately 500 clients. Within the RCCS there were four multidisciplinary case management teams providing, coordinating and monitoring the care of most of the clients in the service. Many of the case managers within these teams were CPNs. In addition there were four teams, again mainly comprising nurses, providing intensive support for clients with secured tenancies in housing association properties or in their own homes.

The present study, conducted in 1990/1991, examined the demographic, psychiatric, service usage, social functioning, problems and service needs of a series of clients referred to RCCS. Information about these clients' own perception of their problems and their quality of life was also col-lected.

Method

Subject. Data were collected on 100 people consecutively referred to RCCS between 1 July 1990 and 26 February 1991. Both those entering the care of the team and those who were rejected by the service or refused service care were considered. Most of these people were referred by the sector CMHTs (88%), but there were also referrals from other specialist teams in the area (e.g. forensic and addiction services).

Data collection and procedure. All clients were identified at the point at which the referral letter was received by RCCS and data were collected from three sources: existing notes and records, the assessing case manager and the client her/himself. Demographic information (age, sex, race, accommodation, occupation, status, etc.), psychiatric history and diagnosis were collected from client notes and team records. Information on social functioning was obtained by the assessing case manager using the Life Skills Profile (Rosen, Hadzi-Pavlovic and Parker, 1989). Information on staff-identified problems and needs was obtained via a semi-structured interview with assessing case managers. Clients were interviewed by the researcher to obtain their views of their problems and needs using an interview format parallel to that employed with case managers. Structured interviews were also conducted with clients to complete the Brief Psychiatric Rating Scale (BPRS, Overall and Gorham, 1962), designed to assess psychiatric symptomatology, and the Quality of Life Assessment.

All information from case managers was obtained within 2 weeks of the team's first assessment of the client. Clients were interviewed in their own homes, given full information about the project and assured that their replies would be confidential and would not affect the care they received. Their participation was, of course, voluntary, but few refused. Of the 100 clients, 80 completed the assessments; the team were unable to contact four of those referred, five refused assessment by the team and were not therefore approached by the researcher, and 11 of those assessed by the team refused to be interviewed by the researcher. Details of the progress of each person referred, including the outcome of the referral and initial services received, were collected from team records.

Results

The RCCS is designed to serve that part of the Nottingham population of long-term mental health service users who are more disabled by their mental health problems. Table 8.2 shows that, while in many ways those referred to RCCS are similar to the entire population of long-term service users in Wandsworth, they fall towards the more disabled end of the spectrum. A higher proportion were single (87%) and none had jobs in open employment. In general, they represented a younger group (mean age 37 years) who nevertheless had a long history of psychiatric problems and the majority had experienced at least one psychiatric hospital admission (92%), although the proportion who had experienced multiple admissions was approximately the same (69% in RCCS referrals, 66% in Wandsworth long-term clients). A higher proportion had a primary diagnosis of schizophrenia (67%) and personality disorder (10%) and fewer had affective disorders. The level of symptomatology (as measured by the BPRS – Overall and Gorham, 1962) was not, on the whole, high, indicating the long-standing and chronic nature of their mental health problems and the importance of social aspects of their disability and care. It is interesting to note that the majority were male – a finding replicated in studies of other specialist rehabilitation and long-term care services (Ford *et al.*, 1993a; Brooker 1994). A substantial proportion had a forensic history or a history of drug/alcohol abuse – characteristics frequently reported in client

Table 8.2 Characteristics of 100 people referred to Nottingham Rehabilitation and Community Care Service

Female (%)	32
Mean age (SD)	37 years (12.0)
Single, divorced, widowed or separated (%)	87
Race/ethnicity (%)	
UK/Irish	93
African Caribbean	4
Asian	3
African	1
Mean no. of years since first contact with psychiatric services (SD)	10.2(8.9)
Mean no. of admissions (SD)	3.5(3.0)
Mean length of longest admission (SD)	12 months (25.0)
Percentage who had spent time in prison	19
Percentage who had spent time in special hospital	13
Primary diagnosis (%)	
Schizophrenia	67
Manic-depressive illness	11
Personality disorder	10
Alcohol/drug dependency	5
Depression	3
Accommodation (%)	
Homeless	10
Supported situation or with family	46
Independent accommodation	28
Psychiatric hospital	12
Occupational status (%)	
In open employment	0
In sheltered work	1
Unemployed	99
Quality of Life mean scores (SD) (all scores out of a possible 6 – higher scores denote higher quality of life)	
Living environment	3.2(1.3)
Family contact and relations	3.1(1.4)
Social contact and relations	2.8(1.3)
Leisure activities	3.0(1.4)
Employment	2.5(1.3)
Finances	0.9(1.6)
Safety	3.8(1.2)
Health	3.8(1.2)
Overall	3.1(1.6)

Table 8.2 *contd*

Brief Psychiatric Rating Scale Scores (mean and SD) – Overall and Gorham, 1962 (all subcategory scores out of a possible 18 – higher scores denote greater symptomatology)	
Thought disturbance	3.9(3.6)
Withdrawal	2.6(2.2)
Anxiety	3.5(2.3)
Hostility	2.2(2.2)
Total	14.1(8.3)
Social functioning (mean standardized scores and SD) – Rosen and Parker, 1989 (higher scores denote poorer functioning)	
Self-care	7.6(0.2)
Non-turbulence (anger control, recklessness, violence, self-harm, etc.)	7.9(0.2)
Social involvement	9.9(0.5)
Communication skills	3.6(0.2)
Responsibility	3.3(0.2)
Outcome of referral (%)	
Not assessed by RCCS	4
Rejected by RCCS	9
Client refused RCCS care	27
Accepted for: day care	31
community residential care	22
outreach case management	7

groups whom services find most challenging to engage and serve (Hirsch *et al.*, 1992; Bachrach, 1982).

Table 8.3 shows that the clients referred, both in their own eyes and in those of their case managers, had multiple problems in a wide range of areas. In both clients' and case managers' opinions, the majority had difficulties in the areas of occupation, frequently reporting being bored and wanting work, and problems with the symptoms of their mental health problems. Others frequently reported problems included housing, loneliness, self-care, finances and relationships. Although side effects of medication have been reported to be a major problem for this client group (Turner, 1993) it is interesting that only 7% of client and 10% of their case managers considered this to be a problem at the time of assessment.

Overall, clients saw themselves as having fewer problems than case managers considered them to have. This is important as people are unlikely to be willing to accept help with difficulties they do not see themselves as having. One of the biggest areas of disagreement arose in the area of 'motivation problems'. Table 8.3 shows that 50% of clients were deemed to have motivation difficulties by their case managers – they showed a lack

Table 8.3 Categories of problems and needs and the number of clients and case managers reporting problems in these areas, including the ranked importance of the categories at baseline

Category	Type of data included	% clients with problems – client's view (rank)	% clients with problems – CM's view (rank)	% agreement between CM and client views of clients' problems
Finance	Large debts or problems budgeting	21(7)	20(8)	82.2
Self-care and domestic skills	Difficulties looking after self, including cooking, self-care, shopping and household tasks	28(5)	41(77)	71.2
Occupation	Boredom through lack of structured activity, or a need/desire to undertake employment training	52(1)	63(2)	68.5
Relationships	Relationship difficulties within family or in living situation and/or poor social skills	25(6)	57(3)	66.3
Loneliness	Lack of friendship, or few social contacts such that client or case manager mention loneliness	41(4)	46(6)	61.5
Motivation	Lack of interest in becoming involved in the service, assertion that they do not want help or do not have problems, or case manager feels that engagement will be difficult because of lack of motivation	21(7)	50(4)	70.3
Medication	Side effects of medication, not taking prescribed medication or feeling that medication is causing problems	7(10)	11(9)	86.3
Mental health	Any symptoms mentioned by clients or case manager as a current problem	50(2)	77(1)	74.0
Medical	Physical disability or illness	12(9)	8(10)	87.7
Housing	Lack of accommodation, inadequate or unsuitable accommodation whether due to insufficient support, untenable relationships within the home or poor physical conditions	42(3)	48(5)	71.2

of interest in or willingness to accept and engage in help and services offered – but only 21% of clients identified such problems. This lack of motivation probably results from the discrepancy between client and staff-identified problems or support needs and poses a challenge to professionals: what to do, for example, when a person has not bathed or changed clothes for several weeks but refuses help in this area, saying s/he has no problems? A total of 41% of clients were identified as requiring help with self-care and domestic chores, while only 28% of clients identified themselves as having problems in these areas. Similarly there was a mismatch between client- and staff-identified problems in the areas of relationship difficulties: most clients described themselves as lonely but not as having the difficulties with relationships or social skills deficits that staff identified in them.

The social functioning of clients (as measured using the Life Skills Profile – Rosen, Hadzi-Pavlovic and Parker, 1989) revealed a wide range of scores in all categories both within and between individuals (see Table 8.2). The worst areas of functioning were in the categories of self-care, disruptive, difficult and reckless behaviour, and social contact. Many were very socially isolated, although interestingly the area of least problems was that of communication skills – suggesting that it is not skills deficits but possibly other factors such as lack of opportunity, stigma, unpredictability and disruptive behaviour that result in social isolation. Interestingly for a group of people who are typically regarded as being unable to take responsibility for themselves this was the area in which these clients showed least disturbance.

One of the most disturbing features of these findings is the poor quality of life reported by those interviewed. On average, scores were around the central point of the scales used indicating that clients had 'mixed feelings' about all areas of their life. The scores show that this group experienced less satisfaction than those reported on similar populations using the same instrument (Simpson, Hyde and Faragher, 1989; Ford *et al.*, 1993a). However the pattern of scores was similar to that found in these other studies with people being most unhappy about their financial situation, work and social opportunities. This poses a dilemma for professionals, who are not always in a position to significantly affect the areas about which clients are most concerned (e.g. the low level of state benefits they receive). However, it is important for professionals to recognize the primary concerns of clients with work, social contacts and finances. Often areas such as work, social contact and explorations of whether an individual can receive all the benefits to which they are entitled receive relatively little attention beside more directly 'clinical' issues.

Table 8.1 shows that, of the 100 people referred, 60 people entered RCCS care: 22 were placed in supported residential settings (some receiving day care as well), and 31 received day care only. All of those in supported accommodation and all but six in day care also received case management services, but a further seven people, generally those who refused other day and residential services, did accept and were accepted for outreach case

Table 8.4 The significant differences between people accepted, rejected and refusing the service

Variable	Accepted (n = 60)	Rejected (n = 9)	Refused (n = 27)	Significance
Living arrangements (%)				$\chi^2 = 21.826\ p < 0.05$
Alone	66.6	33.3	22.2	
With friends	3.3	0	0	
With spouse/cohabitee	10.0	0	29.6	
With parents	23.3	33.3	44.4	
No fixed abode	6.6	22.2	3.7	
Hospital	26.6	11.1	0	
Marital status – % single	90	100	74	$\chi^2 = 5.589\ p < 0.05$
Primary diagnosis (%)				$\chi^2 = 21.222\ p < 0.05$
Schizophrenia	73.3	44.4	62.9	
Affective disorder	15.0	0	18.5	
Anxiety-related	0	0	3.7	
Personality disorder	8.3	44.4	3.7	
Alcohol/drug abuse	1.6	0	7.4	
Other	1.6	11.1	3.7	
Secondary diagnosis (%)				$\chi^2 = 22.888\ p < 0.01$
None	83.3	44.4	77.7	
Schizophrenia	0	0	0	
Affective disorder	0	0	0	
Anxiety-related	1.6	22.2	0	
Personality disorder	1.6	11.1	14.8	
Alcohol/drug abuse	6.6	0	3.7	
Other	6.6	22.2	3.7	
History of drug abuse (%)	20.3	66.6	7.4	$\chi^2 = 5.135\ p = 0.07$
Forensic history (property) (%)	27.1	55.5	25.9	$\chi^2 = 6.154\ p < 0.05$
Spent time in special hospital (%)	10.2	57.1	7.4	$\chi^2 = 13.308\ p < 0.01$
Referrer (%)				$\chi^2 = 21.663\ p < 0.01$
Psychiatrist	55.0	55.5	55.5	
Other mental health worker	41.6	0	37.0	
Self/other	3.3	44.4	7.4	
Approved of referral (%)	78.3	44.4	29.6	$\chi^2 = 9.8452\ p < 0.05$
Knowledge of diagnosis (%)	51.6	33.3	7.4	$\chi^2 = 10.402\ p < 0.05$
Problems/needs (%)				
Client's view				
Medical problems	10.0	33.3	3.7	$\chi^2 = 7.725\ p < 0.05$
Motivation problems	13.3	11.1	29.6	$\chi^2 = 11.685\ p < 0.01$

Table 8.4 *contd*

CM's view				
Housing problems	51.6	44.4	14.8	$\chi^2 = 7.110 \; p < 0.05$
Motivation problems	35.0	33.3	55.5	$\chi^2 = 9.753 \; p < 0.05$
Mean total of admissions (months)	16.5 (SD 30.0)	59.8 (SD 75.3)	13.09 (SD 22.85)	$F_{(2,81)}5.06 \; p < 0.01$
Mean LSP non-turbulence score/36*	6.7 (SD 6.1)	14.7 (SD 8.7)	7.9 (SD 5.2)	$F_{(2,666)}5.47 \; p < 0.01$
Mean total LSP score/117*	30.1 (SD 16.7)	36.9 (SD 21.0)	24.9 (SD 20.4)	$F_{(2,96)}4.42 \; p < 0.01$
Mean QOL score concerning social activity**	2.5 (SD 1.2)	3.5 (SD 0.7)	3.2 (SD 1.1)	$F_{(2,70)}3.16 \; p < 0.05$
Mean QOL score concerning leisure**	3.8 (SD 1.4)	3.8 (SD 1.4)	3.4 (SD 1.3)	$F_{(2,69)}2.59 \; p = 0.08$
Mean QOL score concerning health and service satisfaction**	3.6 (SD 1.2)	2.1 (SD 1.7)	3.9 (SD 0.5)	$F_{(2,65)}4.02 \; p < 0.05$

*Higher score denotes higher levels of problems; **higher score denotes more positive feelings

management only. Of the 40 people referred who were not taken in to RCCS care, four could not be contacted by the RCCS team. Nine were rejected by the RCCS, the reasons typically given being that they were 'too difficult' to be managed in the community-based services offered, although two were considered to be functioning well and therefore not in need of the intensive services offered by RCCS. By far the largest group of the people referred who did not enter RCCS care refused to accept any of the services RCCS offered ($n = 27$). The majority of these people turned down the service once they had seen what was on offer, suggesting that there is some way to go in making services acceptable or attractive to those to whom they are offered. The reasons that clients gave for refusing care would support this assertion, the major problem appearing to lie in identification of and with other clients. The majority of those refusing services felt they would not 'fit in'; they did not see themselves as 'mad' or 'odd', as they perceived the other clients they met to be. Where a client made comments of this type s/he had generally been offered either residential or day care services that necessitated mixing with other service users in a segregated environment. It is a matter for speculation whether such clients would have accepted outreach case management services providing non-stigmatized help and support in the ordinary environments in which they already functioned. Providing help on the clients' terms, rather than on the basis of what professionals think is good for them, can increase uptake of services (Ford *et al.*, 1993b).

The results of a comparison of those who were accepted into RCCS care with those who were rejected and who refused services can be seen in Table 8.4.

Those accepted by the service were likely to be living alone, be single, have a diagnosis of schizophrenia, know their diagnosis and think referral to the RCCS was a 'good idea'. They also tended to have a low level of satisfaction with their social and leisure activities. Overall, these people might best be characterized as a group who recognized their need for support and were receptive to service input.

Those rejected by services ($n = 9$) were all single; two people were homeless and one was hospitalized at the time of referral. They were likely to have a primary diagnosis of personality disorder, multiple diagnoses and histories of drug and alcohol abuse, to have been involved with forensic services and to have spent considerable periods of time in psychiatric hospital. In general, their social functioning was poorer than that of other groups and they often displayed difficult and disruptive behaviour, all indicating that despite their rejection they had considerable need for support and care. They often expressed a poor opinion of psychiatric services and said they were satisfied with their social and leisure activities. Overall, this group of clients showed all the characteristics of rootlessness, 'lack of motivation', denial of difficulties and rejection of help offered which, when combined with challenging behaviour, render them unacceptable to services. They are similar to the group that Hirsch *et al.* (1992) describes as posing 'insoluble problems in the context of modern service provision' despite their high level of support needs Herein lies the challenge to the CPNs who provide much of the outreach care available in Britain today.

Unlike those who were refused by services, those who refused care despite being offered it were similar to those accepted into care except that they were more likely to have a diagnosis of drug/alcohol misuse and a higher level of existing informal support in the community, often from a spouse or parents, possibly reducing their perceived need for alternative 'professional' care. Most said they did not approve of their referral to RCCS or want services. The burden of care on these support networks was not assessed in this study but has been reported elsewhere (Brown, 1985) and also poses problems for service providers.

OVERVIEW OF FINDINGS

These two studies demonstrate the value of thorough assessment of the needs and characteristics of long-term clients as a means of illustrating a variety of factors that are important if CPN services are to adequately target this population. Support for people with such severe and persistent mental health problems is not simply an issue for those working in specialist services specifically targeted at this client group. The first study reported here demonstrates that long-term support and care are a central element of the work of generic community mental health teams, and in particular CPNs, who in most places provide the care for the majority of long-term clients. The second study, conducted in a specialist rehabilitation team, amplifies and

extends the picture of long-term clients' needs and problems and clari-
fies the issues facing those involved in long-term care work, findings that
are important to CPNs whether they work in generic or specialist settings.

These studies both illustrate the challenges that must be met in targeting the needs of people with serious and persistent mental health problems
to ensure that high quality, effective and acceptable services are provided for them. The major findings of these studies can be summarized as
follows.

1. *Ongoing problems arise from long-standing mental health problems.* Many
people who experience long-term and disabling mental health problems require
ongoing treatment and support in social as much as clinical areas. As disabilities
are ongoing, any service must be provided on a non-time-limited basis; as
Bachrach (1982) states, services must have infinite duration and potentially
be available throughout individual patients' lives. Contrary to most traditional
indices of success, discharge or the possibility of discontinuing service input
is not a relevant yardstick of success. Indeed, the converse is probably true:
services might best be judged by their ability to maintain continued input and
contact. Where a person with long-term problems ceases to require service
input, it is important to ensure easy access to support should they require
it again.

2. *Individuals are multiply (but not universally) disabled.* People require
support in a variety of areas, but their personal strengths and aspirations must
not be overlooked. Medication is important, but only as part of a more
comprehensive complex of input and support needs. Many of the supports
that people require fall outside traditional 'professional' roles. Whose job
is it to clean the bath, mow the lawn, take the rent to the rent office or negotiate
with the electricity board? Community care will fail if professionals of all
disciplines, including CPNs, fail to recognize that such apparently mundane
activities are central and critical to maintaining the community tenure of those
who are severely disabled (Stein and Test, 1980). Further, it is clear that
professional jealousies ('this is **my** patient') are destructive to the community
care enterprise. Multiple problems necessitate multiple interventions and
multiple expertise (Bachrach, 1989).

3. *Disabilities are not stable.* Traditionally, rehabilitation theories assumed
a 'ladder' model in which a person was gradually helped to reach her/his
optimal level of functioning and then remained at this level with minimal
support. This is an unfortunate fantasy. Serious mental health problems are
notoriously variable, meaning that a person who one day requires a very low
level of support may the next day require a very high level. It is dangerously

disheartening to both staff and clients if this natural and predictable variability in functioning is construed as failure. All services must continually reassess their clients' needs at any given moment and provide support accordingly; to provide more than is required deskills the client, to provide too little threatens community tenure.

4. *Impairment of functioning in relation to the basic necessities of everyday life* is a major problem for many of this client group. They have problems with basic self-care, nutrition, housing, money – all of which can severely jeopardize community tenure. Poverty in anyone who has to live permanently on state benefits is seriously handicapping. When such poverty has to be negotiated by someone who has difficulty in organizing her/his life it is doubly disabling.

5. *Unemployment and a lack of any meaningful and valued roles and status* is a serious problem. The vast majority of severely disabled people retain a desire to work, to contribute something, yet these studies show that frequently they are denied this. Not only does this severely detract from their quality of life and happiness, but it also has serious negative implications for their mental health: the deleterious effects of unemployment for all of us (whether we have serious mental health problems or not) have been widely documented (Ford, Goddard and Lansdallwelfare, 1987). Further, the specifically deleterious effects of idleness on the negative symptoms of people with serious mental health problems have been highlighted in the classic studies of Wing and Brown (1970).

6. *Social isolation and disrupted social relationships* are a major problem. Most socially disabled people live alone and have few social contacts or activities, and complaints of loneliness and isolation abound. It is ironic that those with serious social disabilities should have less access to the ordinary social contacts, relationships and supports (friends, families, lovers, colleagues) upon which those who are not so disabled rely so heavily. Even where a person does have social contacts these often do not provide the understanding and support that is so necessary; too often those with whom they have contact do not comprehend their problems and mislable them as idle, dangerous, stupid and incompetent (Nunally, 1961; Gove, 1975).

7. *Refusal of/reluctance to accept services*. People with serious mental health problems do not always want what we have to offer; they do not always agree with our assessment of their needs and they may not want to be identified

as mentally ill. Self-concept has been found to be a particular problem among younger, non-institutionalized clients, who identify more strongly with members of the public than with other people who have mental health problems and consequently are reluctant to engage in segregated services for the mentally ill (Thompson, 1988). Problems of drop-out, refusal of services, and the tendency of services to reject those who do not want what they offer and present 'difficult' behaviours, create enormous challenges: how to render services acceptable and attractive to those who need them and how to resist the understandable temptation to give up on those who either are unwilling to accept the care that professionals deem necessary or who do not 'fit in' with what is offered. Often services erect rules like 'we do not accept those with personality disorders'or 'people have to be motivated to change' or 'if you want to come here you have to obey the rules', or less explicitly 'you must accept what we experts think is good for you'. The effect of such written and unwritten policies is to exclude a substantial proportion of people who have a high level of support needs but are unwilling to accept what they are offered.

IMPLICATIONS FOR CPNs

A very large proportion of direct care provided for seriously and persistently mentally ill people in community mental health services is provided by CPNs. The Wandsworth study illustrates that, along with psychiatrists, it is CPNs who provide most input for this group of clients and in the Nottingham RCCS study the majority of case managers were CPNs. Therefore CPNs have a crucial role to play in targeting services to meet the needs of long-term clients. In doing so, they must take into account the specific needs and characteristics of the group. The findings outlined above draw attention to the complexity and importance of this task, facts already recognized by the considerable financial investment made by the Jules Thorn Trust in the development of a national programme of research-based, post-basic education for CPNs, specifically focusing on people with severe and persistent mental illness.

The precedence of social problems and impairment in functioning among these clients demonstrates the importance of practical help, an aspect of care that has historically been undervalued. The move towards nurses specializing in particular forms of therapy represents a move away from the basic necessities of life that are critical to the well-being and community survival of long-term clients. This reinforces the findings of Stein and Test (1980), who demonstrated the potential efficacy of community care for people with severe mental illness. They argued that community care must address all a person's requirements, including material resources (such as food and shelter), coping skills to meet the demands of everyday life, motivation to persevere and remain involved in life, freedom from pathologically dependent relationships, and the support and education of community members involved. This is not a simple task. It involves assessing the individual's needs, abilities and aspirations, analysing where performance is breaking down, designing the most appropriate means of support, maximizing informal supports without over-burdening them and facilitating the most normal, least stigmatizing support methods (for example the use of launderettes and cafes rather than home helps and day centres). All support must be tailored to individual needs and preferences so that care is not only acceptable but appropriate for that person's level of need at that time. Thus the amount of support offered needs to be continually adjusted and titrated to reflect changing levels of functioning. Excessive input may deskill the individual and lead to dependency; insufficient input fails to meet needs, reduces quality of life and may jeopardize community tenure.

The sophistication of the CPN's role with this client group is evidently belied by its frequent characterization as being primarily concerned with giving injections. However, the nurse's role with regard to medication is far from simple; it is a crucial part of the care and treatment package of many clients with severe and persistent mental health problems, involving education of the client and their family, monitoring the effects and side effects of medication, negotiating the most appropriate means of administration for each individual, ensuring regular review and facilitating self-advocacy or advocating on behalf of the client to ensure that their experiences and views are heard and taken into account in the prescription of medication.

Although the challenges posed by this client group demand a pragmatic approach, there is an increasing repertoire of research-based interventions, specifically designed to meet the needs of such clients, that CPNs can draw upon to increase their efficacy in this task. Dominant in these developments is recognition of the client's ability and right to take an active part in their treatment, for example: cognitive–behavioural strategies as a means of coping with and controlling psychotic symptoms (Gardner and Thompson, 1994); education and guidance to facilitate self-monitoring and self-medication as a means of giving clients more control over their lives (Birchwood and Tarrier, 1992); and family interventions based on health education and stress management techniques to improve symptomatology, satisfaction with services and reduce readmissions (Brooker *et al.*, 1993).

Although these approaches reflect an increasing interest in self-help and control, giving people genuine choice does not simply mean presenting options and providing a professional viewpoint. It is a sophisticated exercise in helping people explore what they want and giving them the opportunity to evaluate it. Choice is only meaningful if clients have the right to make bad choices and yet continue to receive support. This involves responsible assessment of risks and the relinquishing of some professional power and control.

Findings from the Nottingham study suggest that 'lack of motivation' is perceived as a major problem by staff endeavouring to provide a service to this client group. A better understanding and a means of helping clients demonstrating apathy, withdrawal, hopelessness and denial of problems is offered by Wing and Morris (1982), and Shepherd (1984) explains such behaviour in terms of 'adverse personal reactions'. These occur when the person finds the idea of mental illness so frightening that s/he cannot accept that s/he has such difficulties and cannot accept the help that is offered – and that may be needed; alternatively, s/he may be so afraid of exacerbatng the symptoms and precipitating further relapse that s/he loses confidence entirely and avoids any stress or challenge. Within this explanation, appropriate intervention would include education and a form of bereavement counselling to facilitate both adaptation to the losses associated with serious mental health problems and realistic recognition of existing potential and strengths.

Although a knowledge of the characteristics and needs of long-term clients enable recommendations to be made regarding the role of CPNs with this client group, there remains the question of targeting those most in need. The Nottingham study suggests that it is the clients least likely to comply with service expectations that are rejected by the service, despite their very high levels of need. This could suggest that services require people to cooperate and be grateful for what is on offer in order to qualify for care. If services were offered on the basis of level of disability, there would be no reason to exclude those people who are 'unable to function at a level expected by themselves, those important to them or society in general' (Wing and Morris, 1982, p. 23) by virtue of their diagnosis or the types of problem they present. However, in order to provide an effective service over long periods of time, CPNs and other service providers need to develop a positive and accepting approach to working with even the most difficult and challenging clients.

Finally, the important issue of clients who refuse services, yet are unable to survive adequately in the community must be addressed. Attractive services that people want to use means services offered on the clients' terms. This remains a challenge to the professionalism of all, including CPNs. Some guidance is offered by the case managers (most of whom were nurses) working specifically with people with severe and persistent mental health problems within the Research and Development for Psychiatry/DoH case management project. After 3 years of case management, 96% of clients accepted for the service remained in contact with appropriate services (Ford *et al.*, 1993b), based on the follow-up of 330 clients; drop-out and refusal of services was therefore minimal. In-depth interviews with clients and case managers suggested that the basis of all this work was the development of long-term, trusting and valuing relationships between workers and clients based on a positive, empathic understanding of the client. Case managers were realistic about the progress that clients could be expected to achieve, yet viewed limited achievements positively through having an understanding of clients' situations and views. A flexible, individualized approach was crucial in allowing clients to set their own goals and persevere with a variety of different strategies over time (Repper, Cooke and Ford, 1993). Perhaps the most important tenet of CPNs' work with people who have severe and persistent mental illness is their own attitude towards these clients. Services are more likely to be appropriate, acceptable, attractive and effective if CPNs are genuinely committed to acknowledging and addressing the needs, rights, aspirations and strengths of the most disabled clients.

REFERENCES

Bachrach, L.L. (1982) Assessment of outcomes in community support systems: results, problems and limitations. *Schizophrenia Bulletin*, **8**, 39–60.

Bachrach, L.L. (1984) De-institutionalisation and women: assessing the consequences of public policy. *American Psychologist*, **39**, 1171–7.

Bachrach, L.L. (1989) The legacy of model programmes. *Hospital and Community Psychiatry*, **40**, 234–5.

Beels, C.C., Gutwirth, L., Berkeley, J. and Struening, E. (1984) Measurement of social support in schizophrenia. *Schizophrenia Bulletin*, **10**, 399–411.

Belcher, R. (1988) Defining the needs of homeless mentally ill persons. *Hospital and Community Psychiatry*, **39**, 1203–5.

Bender, M. and Pilling, S. (1985) A study of variables associated with under-attendance at a psychiatric day centre. *Psychological Medicine*, **15**, 395–401.

Birchwood, M. and Tarrier, N. (1992) *Innovations in the Psychological Management of Schizophrenia. Assessment, Treatment and Services*, John Wiley, Chichester.

Brooker, C.G.D. (1990) A description of clients nursed by community psychiatric nurses whilst attending English National Board Course No. 811: clarification of current role. *Journal of Advanced Nursing*, **15**, 155–6.

Brooker, C. (1994) *British Journal of Psychiatry*, **94**(165), 222–30.

Brooker, C., Tarrier, N., Barrowclough, C. and Butterworth, A. (1993) Skills for CPNs working with seriously mentally ill people: the outcome of a trial of psychosocial intervention, in *Community Psychiatric Nursing: A Research Perspective*, vol. 2, (eds C. Brooker and E. White), Chapman & Hall, London.

Brown, P. (1985) *The Transfer of Care: Psychiatric De-institutionalisation and its Aftermath*, Routledge & Kegan Paul, London.

Coid, J.W. (1988) Mentally abnormal prisoners on remand. 1. Accepted or rejected by the NHS? *British Medical Journal*, **296**, 1779–82.

Dean, C. and Gadd, E.M. (1990) Home treatment for acute psychiatric illness. *British Medical Journal*, **301**, 1021–3.

Department of Health and Social Security (DHSS) (1975) *Better Services for the Mentally Ill*, HMSO, London.

Department of Health and Social Security (DHSS) (1981) *Care in Action*, HMSO, London.

Department of Health (DoH) (1989a) *Caring for People: Community Care into the Next Decade and Beyond*, HMSO, London.

Department of Health (DoH) (1989b) *Discharge of Patients from Hospital*, HC(89)5, HMSO, London.

Department of Health (DOH) (1990a) *NHS and Community Care Act*, HMSO, London.

Department of Health (DOH) (1990b) *The Care Programme Approach for People with a Mental Illness*, HC(90)23, HMSO, London.

Department of Health (DOH) (1990c) *Specific Grant for the Development of Social Services for People with a Mental Illness*, HC(90)24, HMSO, London.

Department of Health (DOH) (1991) *Implementing Community Care*, HMSO, London.

Department of Health (DOH) (1992) *Health of the Nation*, HMSO, London.

Ford, R., Beadsmore, A., Repper, J. *et al.* (1993a) *The Clients and their Needs: Preliminary Results of a Multi-centre Case Management Research Project*, Research and Development for Psychiatry, London.

Ford, R., Beadsmore, A., Repper, J. *et al.* (1993b) *Assertive Outreach for People with Long-term Mental Illness: A Multi-Centre 30 Month Follow-Up Study*, Research and Development for Psychiatry, London.

Ford, M., Goddard, C. and Lansdallwelfare, R. (1987) The dismantling of the mental hospital? Glenside Hospital Surveys 1960–1985. *British Journal of Psychiatry*, **151**, 479–85.

Gardner, B. and Thompson, S. (1994) Strategic thinking. *Nursing Times*, **90**, 32–4.

Gove, W.L. (1975) Labelling mental illness: a critique, in *The Labelling of Deviance*, (ed. W.L. Gove), John Wiley, New York.

Hirsch, S., Craig, T., Dean, C. *et al.* (1992) *Facilities and Services for the Mentally Ill with Persisting Severe Disabilities*, Working Party Report on Behalf of the Royal College of Psychiatrists, Royal College of Psychiatrists, London.

Holloway, F., Davies, G., Silverman, M. and Wainwright, T. (1988) How many beds? A survey of needs for treatment and care in an inpatient treatment unit. *Bulletin of the Royal College of Psychiatrists*, **11**, 398–407.

Hoult, J. and Reynolds, I. (1983) Psychiatric hospital versus community treatment; the results of a randomised trial. *Australian and New Zealand Journal of Psychiatry*, **17**, 160–7.

Jenkins, J. (1989) Nottingham needs assessment planning project survey. Planning Department, Mapperley Hospital, Nottingham, unpublished paper.

Johnstone, E.C., Owens, D.G.C., Gold, A. *et al.* (1984) Schizophrenic patients discharged from hospital – a follow-up study. *British Journal of Psychiatry*, **145**, 586–90.

Jones, K., Robinson, M. and Golightly, M. (1986) Long-term psychiatric patients in the community. *British Journal of Psychiatry*, **149**, 537–40.

Knapp, M., Cambridge, P., Thomason, C. *et al.* (1990) *Care in the Community: Lessons from a Demonstration Programme*, PSSRU, University of Kent, Canterbury.

Koran, M., Sox, H.C., Marton, K.I. *et al.* (1989) Medical evaluation of psychiatric patients 1: Results in a state mental health system. *Archives of General Psychiatry*, **46**, 733–40.

Lehman, A.F., Ward, N. and Linn, L. (1982) Chronic mental patients: the quality of life issue. *American Journal of Psychiatry*, **139**, 1271–6.

Meltzer, D., Hale, S., Malik, S.J. *et al.* (1991) Community care for patients with schizophrenia one year after hospital discharge. *British Medical Journal*, **303**, 1023–6.

Milner, G. (1991) Worcester development project; the closure and replacement of a mental hospital. *Health Trends*, 4, 141–5.
Nunally, J. (1961) Evaluation of treatment effectiveness in psychiatric research. *British Journal of Psychiatry*, 152, 696–8.
O'Driscoll, C., Marshall, J. and Reed, J. (1990) Chronically ill patients in a District General Hospital unit. A survey and two year follow-up in an inner London health district. *British Journal of Psychiatry*, 157, 694–792.
Olfsen, M. (1990) Assertive community treatment: evaluation of the experimental evidence. *Hospital and Community Psychiatry*, 41, 634–41.
Overall, J.E. and Gorham, D.R. (1962) The brief psychiatric rating scale. *Psychological Medicine*, 10, 799–812.
Perkins, R. and Dilks, S. (1992) Worlds apart: working with severely disabled people. *Journal of Mental Health*, 1, 3–17.
Perkins, R. and Rowland, L. (1986) *Community Focussed Psychiatric Services for People with Major Long Term Needs*, District Services Centre/National MIND Joint Conference, Institute of Psychiatry, London.
Prevost, J.A. (1989) Youthful chronicity: paradox of the 1980s. *Hospital and Community Psychiatry*, 33, 173.
Reed, J. (1991) The future of psychiatry, *Psychiatric Bulletin*, 15, 396–401.
Repper, J., Cooke, A. and Ford, R. (1993) How can nurses build trusting relationships with people who have severe and long term mental health problems? Experiences of case managers and their clients. *Journal of Advanced Nursing*, in press.
Rosen, A., Hadzi-Pavlovic, D. and Parker, G. (1989) The Life Skills Profile: a measure assessing function and disability in schizophrenia. *Schizophrenia Bulletin*, 15, 325–37.
Sayce, L., Craig, T. and Boardman, A. (1991) The development of community mental health centres in the UK. *Social Psychiatry and Psychiatric Epidemiology*, 26, 14–20.
Shepherd, G. (1984) *Institutional Care and Rehabilitation*, Longman, New York.
Showalter, E. (1987) *The Female Malady*, Virago, London.
Simpson, C.J., Hyde, C.E. and Faragher, E.G. (1989) The chronically mentally ill in community facilities: a study of quality of life. *British Journal of Psychiatry*, 154, 77–82.
Stein, L. and Test, M.A. (1980) Alternatives to mental hospital treatment. *Archives of General Psychiatry*, 37, 392–7.
Thapa, K. and Rowland, L. (1989) Quality of life perspectives in long-term care: staff and patient perceptions. *Acta Psychiatrica Scandinavica*, 80, 267–71.
Thompson, E.H. (1988) Variation in the self-concept of young adult chronic patients: youthful chronicity re-considered. *Hospital and Community Psychiatry*, 39, 260–4.
Timms, P.W. and Fry, A.H. (1989) Homelessness and mental illness. *Health Trends*, 21, 71–2.
Turner, G. (1993) Client/CPN contact during administration of depot medications: implications for practice, in *Community Psychiatric Nursing: A Research Perspective*, vol. 2, (eds C. Brooker and E. White), Chapman & Hall, London.
Warden, A., Walsh, A. and Becker, S. (1990) *Sentenced to Live Within That Sickness: Mental Health, Social Security and Registered Homes*, Benefits

Research Unit, Nottingham University in association with Nottinghamshire Welfare Rights Service, Nottingham.

Weller, M. (1989) Psychosis and destitution at Christmas 1985–1988. *Lancet*, **ii**, 1509–11.

Wells, K.B., Stewart, A., Hays, R.D. *et al.* (1989) The functioning and well being of depressed patients: results from the medical outcomes study. *Journal of the American Medical Association*, **262**, 914–19.

White, E. (1993) Community psychiatric nursing 1980–1990: a review of organisation, education and practice, in *Community Psychiatric Nursing: A Research Perspective*, vol. 2, (eds C. Brooker and E. White), Chapman & Hall, London.

Wing, J.K. (1982) Course and prognosis of schizophrenia, in *Handbook of Psychiatry, vol 3. Psychoses of Uncertain Aetiology*, (eds J.K. Wing and L. Wing) Cambridge University Press, Cambridge.

Wing, J.K. and Brown, G.W. (1970) *Institutionalism and Schizophrenia*, Cambridge University Press, Cambridge.

Wing, J.K. and Morris, B. (1981) Clinical basis of rehabilitation, in *Handbook of Psychiatric Rehabilitation Practice*, (ed. J.K. Wing), Oxford University Press, Oxford.

Wooff, K. and Goldberg, D.P. (1988) Further observations on the practices of CPNs in Salford: differences between community psychiatric nurses and mental health social workers. *British Journal of Psychiatry*, **153**, 30–7.

CHAPTER NINE

Community psychiatric nurses in relation to diversion schemes

Lisa Maclean

INTRODUCTION

Recently there has been a shift of emphasis in managing the offender with mental health problems. It has become apparent after research (Joseph, 1992; Gunn, 1991; Dell and Robertson, 1993) that it is not always appropriate for the mentally disordered offender to navigate the legal process, which may culminate in their inappropriate imprisonment. The White Paper *The Health of the Nation* (Department of Health, 1992) stated that 'mentally disordered people who commit offences are a particularly vulnerable group. There is a risk that if their health and social care needs are not met they may slip into a vicious circle of offending, imprisonment, reoffending and deteriorating mental health'.

A mentally disordered offender is defined by Reed (1992) as 'mentally disordered person who has broken the law. In identifying broad service needs, this term is sometimes loosely used to include mentally disordered people who are alleged to have broken the law'. Mustill (1991) defines the term 'mentally disordered offender' as an artificial construct, not corresponding to any objectively determinable section of the population. Those suffering from psychiatric disorders or learning disabilities and, in some cases, those who have committed sexual offences seem to come within the remit of diversion schemes for mentally disordered offenders.

Although throughout recent history the mentally disordered offender (MDO) has been managed differently from the 'ordinary offender', the latest initiative of diverting the mentally disordered offender from the criminal justice process is seen as a radical change, and at the 'cutting edge' of this change is the community psychiatric nurse's (CPN's) involvement with the diversion process.

In the late Middle Ages it was established that it was unlawful to imprison someone if s/he was 'mentally disordered' (Reed, 1992). The Vagrancy Act of 1744 made the distinction between impoverished 'lunatics' and 'rogues, vagabonds, sturdy beggers and vagrants'. They were ordered to be detained in a secure place. From the early nineteenth century provision for 'criminal lunatics' and 'lunatics' developed along different lines, though in both cases they were in institutions or custodial care.

The Percy Commission was set up in the 1950s and reported that there should be new emphasis towards community care, with the breaking down of barriers between the mentally ill, mentally handicapped and the general population (Percy Commission, 1957). This led to the Mental Health Act 1959, which replaced legislation dating back to the last century on criminal lunacy and mental deficiency.

The Butler Committee of 1975 (Butler Report, 1975) was set up to look at the specific needs of mentally disordered offenders. It concluded that:

> The overriding need is to provide the best possible treatent for the patients' mental disorder. They should have full access to treatment in the best location that will suit their needs. Ultimately in individual cases this must depend on clinical judgement, but in general policy we hope that humane counsels will prevail, and that considerations of a patient's background will not be allowed to obscure that basic principle.

Butler recommended provision of 2000 secure units with lower levels of security than special hospitals. At the same time, the Glancy working party (Glancy, 1974) was addressing the needs of those already in hospital. These joint recommendations produced the Medium or Regional Secure Units, although these now only provide 600 beds, substantially fewer than both Butler and Glancy recommended.

In 1987, following the 1983 Mental Health Act, the Department of Health/ Home Office Working Group made recommendations for the smoother transfer of MDOs from the prison system to the NHS. In 1989, the Special Hospitals Service Authority took over the management of high-security psychiatric provision from the Department of Health. At the same time there was a growth in community care services, with the emphasis on closure of large institutions.

Even in the 1990s, the Parliamentary Secretary for Health was concerned for the welfare of mentally disordered offenders, as they were still unsuitably placed within the prison system or in high security regimes, when they should have been in hospital.

The majority of offences committed by mentally disordered people have tended to be minor in nature (Coids, 1988) (for example, stealing small items of food and shelter) arising from underlying mental disturbance or lack of care or support. Similarly, the criminal justice system may not know that offenders have already had treatment from the local psychiatric services. Prison is not an appropriate place for most MDOs; indeed it can lead to an exacerbation of their condition (Pitt, 1993). The efficiency scrutiny of the prison medical service (Woolfe and Tumin, 1990) proposed that health care should be contracted into the prisons. This was based on the Woolfe report on disturbances in Manchester Prison and its recommendations for the improvement of prison regimes. Gunn's (1991) research into mentally disordered prisoners suggested that upwards of 700 sentenced prisoners might require transfer to psychiatric care in NHS hospitals.

Given the above, the diversion of some mentally disordered offenders from the criminal justice system and the planning of more appropriate alternative resources have been given priority. In 1990 the Home Office issued Circular 66/90, which promoted the diversion and discontinuance mechanisms to ensure that offenders did not get caught up in the legal system when it was not warranted. The need to divert was derived from two main factors: the negative factors associated with inappropriate imprisonment and the overcrowding of prisons and the positive factor of intervening early enough to prevent the offender from becoming involved in a long pattern of reoffending (recividism), thus giving him/her access to health care provision.

The Reed Committee was set up in 1991 to review the existing services available and make recommendations for future provision.

The Reed review particularly addressed:

1. the level and range of provision that needed to be in place to enable the mentally disordered offender and similar patients to receive care and treatment in the most suitable location;
2. the mechanisms that would:
    (a) estimate the numbers needing specialized services;
    (b) identify and assess the needs of those who should be diverted before entry into the criminal justice system or as soon as possible thereafter;
    (c) ensure effective joint working between the range of agencies locally . . . and government departments nationally;
    (d) make the best use of available resources and ensure that there were no disincentives or unnecessary obstacles to providing the most effective care.

The guiding principles for the service provision were that patients should be cared for:

1. with regard to the quality of care and proper attention to needs of individuals;
2. as far as possible in the community, rather than in institutional settings;
3. under conditions of no greater security than was justified by the degree of damage they presented to themselves or to others;
4. in such a way as to maximize rehabilitation and their chances of sustaining an independent life;
5. as near as possible to their own homes or families if they had them.

Government policy clearly reflected the view that wherever possible mentally disordered offenders should be diverted from the criminal justice system and dealt with by health and social services. The task therefore was to develop the practice of diversion in order to provide the best and most effective response to mentally disordered offenders, while at the same time ensuring the public were adequately protected (NACRO, 1991a). NACRO defined the term 'diversion' as a process of decision making that resulted in certain offenders not being prosecuted but being responded to differently (NACRO, 1991a).

There are now opportunities for diverting the MDO from prosecution at different stages of the criminal justice process. Decisions to divert at a particular stage will depend on the nature and degree of the mental disturbance and the seriousness of the alleged offence. CPNs are involved in all stages of the diversion process.

For the purposes of this chapter, the term 'CPN' will be used when discussing the role of the nurse within diversion schemes. However, it should be noted that not all nurses working in this area have this title and other terms used are, for example, forensic community psychiatric nurse (FCPN), community forensic psychiatric nurse (CFPN), registered mental nurse (RMN), mentally disordered offender scheme nurse (MENDOS nurse) and project workers. The involvement of the CPN in diversion schemes is not entirely the result of Circular 66/90 and the Reed Report (1992) although Reed's identification of a role for nurses in such schemes has undoubtedly resulted in more nurses being appointed.

Prior to the publication of these documents, nurses working in secure units identified a lack of provision for their clients on discharge. Attempts were made to resolve this, with staff from the secure units providing follow-up work (Higgins, 1991; Burrows, 1993). Such activity was apparent in the mid 1980s (Loo, 1984), and even in the late 1970s (Pederson, 1980).

AIM

The aim of this study was to explore the role of a diversion scheme CPN. To do this, it was necessary to pinpoint the CPN's role within the diversion in schemes being set up around the country. There is a paucity of literature relating to the nurse's role, so there has been some reliance on anecdotal evidence based on one-to-one interviews and discussions with nurses working in this area.

To effectively meet the aim it was necessary to review the following questions.

1. Why divert mentally disordered offenders from the criminal justice system?
2. Are diversion schemes meeting needs?

3. Why and how are nurses being employed to facilitate the running of the diversion schemes?
4. What skills do CPNs need to fulfil this role?

METHOD

From the outset, it was apparent that there was a paucity of literature on diversion schemes and even less on the CPN's role in diversion schemes. The literature upon which this chapter has been based was accessed in two ways:

1. a library-based literature search using manual and electronic information sources (e.g. CD-ROM);
2. direct contact with nurses working in the area, requesting any unpublished or locally published reports and other documents.

The search used two university libraries and one hospital library. This gave immediate access to a broad range of indices, bibliography/abstract sources and journals. A strict timescale was not placed on the search, though the period from the mid-1980s to the present was thought to be most relevant. However, library technology sources such as CD-ROM allow rapid and efficient literature searching and therefore, in the area of electronic information, the search was extended back into the 1970s.

The search required a range of different key terms. Preferred key terms differed considerably between different abstracts, journals and indices. For example, Medline preferred 'mentally disordered offender' and Psychlit stored the equivalent information under 'mentally ill offender'. CD-ROM technology allowed for experimentation with key terms (e.g. 'offender' and 'nurse') and assisted the user by providing indexes of key terms and a more in-depth thesaurus. In general, the nursing bibliographies and abstracting journals required less specific terms. The following terms were found to be helpful in conducting the search: mentally disordered offender, mentally abnormal offender, inmate, mentally ill inmate, prison nursing, diversion (and combinations of such terms).

The following sources were used.

Nursing Bibliographies. This represented a selection of key material received by the Royal College of Nursing. It mainly included British journal articles, some books, theses and reports, though international material deemed to be pertinent to British nursing was included. A total of 285 journals contributed abstracts to this source. A particular problem with *Nursing Bibliographies* was that it was updated at a much slower pace than other abstracting sources. Article abstracts did not appear in the bibliographies for at least a year following their publication. Both *Popular Medical Index* (Lister Hospital) and *National Medical Index* (Poole General Hospital) were more up to date, though neither was specific to nursing and both include fewer journals. ASSIA (*Applied Social Sciences Index and Abstracts*) covered English language journals and a broad range of subjects including sociology and psychology. ASSIA is available on CD-ROM, but not at the search sites used for this study.

Electronic information sources. While a manual search should not be avoided, a far more extensive search can be carried out using CD-ROM, including CINAHL (*Cumulative Index to Nursing and Allied Health*), which holds 3200 international, particularly English-language, nursing and allied health journals, is updated quarterly and covers the period 1983 to present; Medline, which also holds 3200 journals, mainly English-language, with English abstracts of some foreign language journals – it is possible to extend the search as far back as 1966; and Psychlit, which covers 1300 journals (international, mainly English-language) from 1974 to the present (books and chapters of books are also stored). Both Medline and Psychlit are updated monthly.

Direct contact literature search. Because of the poverty of available information on the CPN's role in diversion schemes in the above sources, the literature search scope was broadened to include unpublished papers and papers in preparation, scheme newsletters, handouts and working documents. This literature could only be accessed by personal contact with nurses and other professionals involved in diversion schemes.

FINDINGS

Why divert mentally disordered offenders from the criminal justice system?

In recent years there has been growing concern about the treatment of people with mental disorder/health problems being dealt with by the criminal justice system (Sadler, 1989; Dell and Robertson, 1993; McMillan, 1993; Shaw and Simpson, 1991; Coids, 1988; Gunn, 1991), although it is important to note that the concern about mentally disordered offenders is not a recent phenomenon. Staite and Martin (1993) cite the surgeon of Newgate jail, as early as 1835, repeatedly complaining about the number of 'insane' inmates in his charge. Indeed, the criminal justice system in England and Wales has continued to be slow to recognize the needs of those with mental health problems.

English law has, until relatively recently, only considered mental disorder in terms of fitness to plead or awareness of wrong doing (Shaw and Simpson, 1991).

The only defence open to a mentally ill person was to establish a causal link between their 'illness' and the offence. Insanity, madness and lunacy are imprecise concepts and have different meanings from the legal and medical perspectives (Freeman and Roesch, 1989). After the trial of Daniel

McNaughton in 1843, insanity was defined in English Common Law. McNaughton was acquitted of murder with a special verdict of 'not guilty by reason of insanity'. At the time, there was no agreement that the concept of mental incapacity was a defence against crime. The rules of 'insanity' were then formulated by the Law Lords; these have become known as the 'McNaughton Rules':

> Every man is presumed to be sane and to possess a sufficient degree of reason to be responsible for his crimes until the contrary is proved to the satisfaction of the jury and that to establish a defence on the grounds of insanity it must clearly be proved that, at the time of committing the act, the accused was labouring under such defect of reason, from disease of mind, as not to know he was wrong doing
>
> (West and Walker, 1977)

The basis for these rules is the concept of 'knowing'. Unfortunately, what someone else knows is a mystery, and opinions are subjective. Decisions about the degree of responsibility of a defendant can differ among psychiatrists and the jury alike. To illustrate this, Gunn (1981) pointed out that it was legally possible for the defendant to be: mentally normal and insane; mentally disordered and insane; mentally disordered and fully responsible.

The insanity defence has troubled psychiatrists because it has been the sole mechanism by which an offender could be admitted to hospital rather than to prison.

Similarly, it is seen as unjust to make a mentally disordered offender the subject of a criminal trial (Gostin, 1984) if he is unable to comprehend the proceedings and contribute to his own defence. It would be unfair to convict such a person because, if he were capable, he might be able to clear himself of blame. Mental disorder may substantially reduce a defendant's ability to testify, to recall exonerating circumstances or identify corroborative witnesses, to instruct his lawyer, and so forth. Also, he may be highly suggestible, even to the point of incriminating himself when he is not in fact guilty.

The Mental Health Act 1959 was introduced to try and deal with some of these issues and the search for a solution continued with the Mental Health Act 1983. The 1959 Mental Health Act was seen as a complex and enlightened piece of legislation which contained a new notion of voluntary treatment, or 'care without compulsion'. This allowed a hospital order to be made for an offender, without the necessity for proof of a link between mental disorder and the offence. The Act recognized four forms of mental disorder: mental illness, mental impairment, severe mental impairment and psychopathic disorder.

The expectation was that the MDO would receive different treatment from the 'normal offender', i.e. therapy as opposed to punishment. However, in the view of Gostin (1984), there had been insufficient consideration of the comparative effects of a hospital order and a prison sentence. The objective for a mentally disordered offender admitted to hospital is that they should receive treatment. It should also be realized, however, that there is an element of punishment in any judicial decision to confine an individual involuntarily. Although a hospital has an essential caring function, compulsory admission is often just as much a deprivation of liberty as a prison sentence.

The main advantage of a hospital over prison is that it does not represent public control, or at least it is a more subtle version of it. The offender in hospital is treated according to his behaviour, with less loss of personal identity and self respect than can occur in prison (Black, 1984). However, if an offender is admitted to a special hospital or secure unit s/he is subject to the same security as in prison, with the attempt to provide treatment, which is essentially voluntary, taking place under conditions of control associated with a sentence. This can cause problems when, for example, the offender reaches the rehabilitative stage of treatment and his/her need to experience normal activities is curtailed by the restricted environment (Black, 1984).

If the mentally disordered offender is admitted to hospital and cannot be treated, confinement is likely to be of indefinite duration (Gostin, 1984). Therefore, the sentence served may prove longer than the period of imprisonment that would be expected if the MDO was 'punished' instead of treated (Higgins, 1991; Joseph, 1992).

If there is uncertainty about the length of confinement, because of the expected or desired changes in the individual's character and affect necessary to satisfy others before returning to society, this may result in a deep sense of unfairness and may ultimately be countertherapeutic.

The duration of the hospital order should be proportionate to the gravity of the offence and should not be greater than the period of time the offender would spend in prison.

> It may be right for society to protect itself under certain circumstances against particular individuals who have clearly demonstrated that they can be destructive, but if we are to detain people much longer than we would otherwise punish them then we must establish proper rules for doing this and allow plenty of opportunity for an appeal against that decision. Justice is justice whether the recipient is bad, mad or both.
>
> (Gunn, 1979)

The 1959 Mental Health Act was intended to result in the removal of large numbers of MDOs from prison and make for easier disposal for the courts. However, at the same time during the late 1950s and 1960s, there were developments to integrate patients with the lives of others in the community. New drugs became available that could control bizarre behaviour and there was more awareness of the effects of institutionalism (Barnum, 1992). The spirit of the Act was to ensure that the psychiatric patients should, as far as possible, be treated no differently from physically ill patients. Thus, there was the development of 'informal' admission, outpatients departments, day hospitals, and so forth.

There was an increasing 'open door' policy in most psychiatric hospitals; large numbers of long-stay patients were being transferred into the community. Admissions to hospital were shorter, patients were being discharged more quickly and this gave rise to the 'revolving door patient'. Chronically ill patients came to be seen by staff as 'bed-blockers' (Gostin, 1984). Patients who were violent, or unsettled, were refused by 'open door' hospitals. Instead, they were redirected towards secure provision such as prison (Neilson, 1992; Hoggett, 1990).

Once the secure provision became overcrowded, alternatives had to be found. The Glancy report (1974) and the Butler report (1975) addressed the issue of separate provision for mentally disordered offenders. Specifically, Butler recommended medium-secure provision, which offered an alternative to local psychiatric hospitals and special hospitals, and also the development of community-based forensic psychiatric services. It would seem that these recommendations have still not been fully implemented, as Courtney and Cunnane (1992) confirmed that there is still a lack of long-stay provision in secure units. Thus, many offenders still find themselves within the prison system.

Research in recent years (Coids, 1988) has indicated that offending by those who suffer from mental disorder is often related to social circumstances resulting from the mental disorder and/or from lack of support in the community. Many offenders are convicted of petty offences (Coids, 1988) that are committed without planning or skill, e.g. theft of food or small amounts of money. Such offences are motivated by basic needs. In these cases it is impossible to say with confidence that the offender would not have committed the offence if he had not been mentally disordered (Walker and McCabe, 1973). Robertson (1988) compared the justice system to the practice of fishing with a net. This net 'catches a disproportionate number of clumsy, inept or incompetent men; the result is that the mentally ill in the community are bound to be over represented'. The report of Gunn (1991) on the numbers of those with psychiatric disorders among the sentenced and remand population lend support to this view.

Pitt (1993) reported appalling conditions within prisons, which are arguably inhumane for any inmate but all the more so for those suffering from mental health problems. He described those assessed to be of self-harm or suicidal risk as often housed in awful conditions (alone, without supervision) stripped and put in a canvas suit. He felt that such conditions exacerbated the mental health condition. There is a high psychiatric morbidity reported among prisoners (Gunn, 1991). Woolfe (1991) indicated that mentally ill inmates could not cope with the prison regimes and required extra attention at the expense of other prisoners. Morrison's study (Morrison, 1991) revealed that mentally ill inmates, who were dependent and lacked social and economic resources, were more vulnerable to victimization by other inmates. There has also been criticism of prison hospitals. Gunn (1991) reported that often patients were confined in conditions that outside prison would cause 'public outcry'.

Prisons are seen as costly and unnecessary for the 'inadequate offender' (Lawson, 1984). For the minority who, on the grounds of dangerousness, do need special hospital/prison care, the secure milieu should also be constructive, humane and caring. At the very least, it should not cause a person to return to the community more brutalized than when s/he came in. Over-crowded special hospitals belatedly raised their criteria for admission and refused to take some offenders on the grounds that they were not difficult or dangerous enough to warrant their high security facilities. Courts began to experience increasing difficulties in finding a bed for clearly mentally ill defendants as mental hospitals refused them on the grounds that they were too difficult/untreatable or both (Gostin, 1984). Mentally disordered offenders have been very low in the priorities of government departments, the health service and the criminal justice system (Bluglass, 1993). Both Barnum (1992) and Hoggett (1990) support this view and make particular reference to the National Health Service's reluctance to make provision for mentally disordered offenders; Barnum comments that the recent health service reforms provide 'ample' financial disincentives to make such provision. Mental disorder is in itself not sufficient justification for admission to hospital, as some mental disorders can be coped with adequately without admission. Similarly defend-ants should not simply receive custodial care in hospital. It is important that hospitals are not used for the purpose of prevention or to begin a period of confinement, and that scarce resources in the health service are not allocated to people who cannot benefit from treatment.

A change in such prioritizing was given impetus by the Butler report (1975) and more recently by Home Office Circular 66/90 (Home Office, 1990), which emphasized the need to divert the mentally disordered offender from the criminal justice system to the care of the health and or social services, together with the Reed report (1992), which placed much emphasis on the need for multi-agency working with this client group. A number of schemes aimed at diverting the mentally disordered offender from the criminal justice system were set up, seemingly in direct response to Circular 66/90 and the Reed report.

Is diversion effective?

The government's document *The Health of the Nation* (Department of Health, 1992) expressed concern that mentally disordered offenders were a particularly vulnerable group and were liable to become trapped in a cycle of offence, imprisonment, increasing disability from their mental illness and then, on release, a further offence.

The Home Office Circular 66/90 (Home Office, 1990) and the Reed report (Reed, 1992) addressed this specific issue and provided an impetus for the emergence of multi-agency diversion schemes that attempt to divert such offenders before conviction. These schemes work with the offender while on remand, in court and even at the point of arrest, or soon after.

The Criminal Justice Act 1991 made changes for the provision of mentally disordered offenders, by opening up the options available. For example, it made pre-sentence reports mandatory before custody and required the court to order a medical report if the offender appeared to be mentally disordered, as well as to consider the effect of custody on the mental condition and any treatment available for it (Dobson, 1992).

Reed (1992) made 276 recommendations in all. The report set the following guiding principles: there should be proper attention to the needs of the individual, as far as possible in the community rather than in an institutional setting, and under conditions of no greater security than was required by the degree of danger presented by the offender. In addition, maximum opportunity was to be sought for rehabilitation and the chance of sustaining an independent life for the individual as near as possible to his/her own home or family.

Early diversion of those with mental disorder from the criminal justice system encapsulated all those principles. Reed recommended that diversion schemes should be set up to be relevant to the needs of each individual locality. The main implication for patients was that they should not be disadvantaged by their status as offenders.

Reed's main emphasis, however, was on multi-agency working. Cheswick (1992) agreed with this principle, but thought that it might be difficult to facilitate as agencies were already struggling with new funding arrangements and new roles. The Department of Health (1992) requested the regional directors of public health to regularly assess the needs of their clients for secure provision and for non-secure places for those suffering from mental disorder. It was emphasized that this should be a cooperative operation with all agencies involved in the management and diversion of mentally disordered offenders. This activity should become a regular joint agency activity that would keep the service under review, as this would enhance the coordinated approach to the care of this client group (Jones and Dean, 1992).

It was acknowledged by Reed that local secure and community provision required assessment. Such assessment needed to take into account not only early diversion but also provision for MDOs who had been incarcerated on their release from prison. The results of this assessment needed to be incorporated into local community care philosophies and into the contracting arrangements between purchasers and providers.

The perceived aims of a diversion scheme would therefore seem to be threefold: firstly to provide for a more humanitarian disposal of the mentally disordered offender (Cooke, 1992; Dell and Robertson, 1993); secondly to reduce recividism ('revolving door syndrome') (Stuart-White, 1991); and thirdly to reduce the cost of inappropriate imprisonment (James and Hamilton, 1991).

It would appear from the literature that there is little dispute that diversion from custody, where appropriate provision has been made, is more humane. Whether or not diversion has an impact on recidivism and cost is far from clear.

With regard to recidivism, it is hard to tell from the available literature whether diverting the mentally disordered offender reduces the likelihood of re-offending. Rice and Harris (1992) made a comparison of recidivism among schizophrenic and non-schizophrenic offenders. They found that the schizophrenic group were less likely to reoffend than the non-schizophrenic group. While Rice and Harris drew no firm conclusions as to why this might be, they noted that their non-schizophrenic offender subjects were more likely to have a history of alcohol abuse and be under the influence of alcohol at the time of the offence. Cooke's (1992) study on recidivism at the Douglas Inch Centre produced similar findings – that there was a positive relationship between alcohol and substance addiction and re-offending. Rice and Harris (1992) suggested that, in addition to the above, the lower recidivism among schizophrenics may be evidence of good clinical practice in terms of effective treatment and decisions about discharge. However, they stressed the need for a focus on those factors related to the commission of criminal behaviour as well as treatment of the specific mental disorder. The findings of both Cooke (1992) and Robertson (1988) would tend to support this.

With regard to cost, James and Hamilton (1991, 1992) suggest that earlier assessment of mentally disordered offenders might significantly reduce cost. Such offenders spend less time on remand. Where a hospital order was made, this would be completed at an earlier stage and this suggested the possibility of an improved prognosis and shortened overall stay in hospital. So, instead of a straight transfer of cost from the prison to the health system, the cost to the prison service is removed altogether and the cost to the health service is substantially reduced. Johnson and Smith (1993) considered that the cost of specialist provision for the mildly mentally handicapped offender was 'not cheap' and that arguably imprisonment, in the short term, was less expensive. However Reed (1992) pointed out that this particular group was likely to be very small. It could equally be argued that the new demands made on hospitals, community care and the courts could result in an increase in the cost of managing this client group (Hedderman, 1993).

At present, the effectiveness of diversion schemes rests upon evidence that is largely anecdotal. Such schemes are still in their infancy and data have not yet been fully collated. However, the results of the diversion scheme at Bournville Lane Police Station, Birmingham (diversion at, or just after, arrest) were published in a practitioner's newsletter, and are an initial indication of how the scheme is working. A total of 336 people were screened, which represented 19.16% of the cases through the custody suite. Of these, 25 were identified as having a mental health problem (7.44% of the people screened). Of those with mental health problems, 16 were identified routinely by the CPN and nine, after referral, by the police, most usually by the custody sergeant. The most common form of behaviour leading to a referral was verbal aggression and damage to property. Of those identified, 48% were already known to the psychiatric services through inpatient or outpatient psychiatric care services. In 14 of the 25 cases, the police immediately dropped all the charges. Of the remainder, five were released into the community on police bail; six were remanded in custody. Of the 14 immediately diverted at the point of arrest, two were admitted informally and three under compulsory admission (Section 2 of the Mental Health Act 1983) to general psychiatric care. Three were referred as outpatients to the regional secure unit, three as outpatients to the general services and one to a day care centre (Spurgeon, 1993).

This report and much anecdotal evidence does suggest that people are being effectively intercepted and screened for mental health problems using these models of diversion. It also highlights the reduced burden on the prison system brought about by the opportunity for early intervention and assessment for any mental health problems.

There could be a clash of philosophies when MDOs are diverted at the pre-court stage. If, in treating offenders, the assumption is made that they should be responsible for their own actions, where does it leave people who may see themselves as being excused because they are/were ill at the time of the offence? Does diversion really help them, or is it patronizing and merely confirms that they are unable to cope? Diversion may also remove their opportunity of disproving in court the allegations made against them. Moreover, where does it leave the victims? Without a conviction there is no access to the Criminal Justice Board and courts cannot order compensation (Griffiths, 1993).

The crucial question to be addressed is, what provision is made for mentally disordered offenders **after** diversion? The need to develop services beyond the point of diversion is essential. Little information is available about what happens to those who have been diverted from the criminal justice process, but it seems probable that many of their health and social care needs go unmet, making it more likely that they will experience recurring mental ill health or re-offend (NACRO, 1991a). It is important that diversion schemes do not become another revolving door service. Resources need to be made available to support people in the community, giving them access to housing and practical support. The recent Clunis report (Home Office, 1994) showed that there needs to be follow-up, particularly of clients who are seen as being dangerous to themselves or others.

Examples of innovations in provision for mentally disordered offenders can be found in Hertfordshire and the West Midlands. The CPN in the Hertfordshire scheme was involved in setting up a day centre provision for MDOs, called CHIPS (Community Health Integrated Programme Services). CHIPS provided follow-up care after discharge into the community, enabling such clients to stabilize and integrate back into society. Everall (1993) reported that CHIPS helped to create a forum for, and culture of, peer support among its attenders.

In the West Midlands there has been a project to develop bail hostels specifically for 'diverted' offenders. As the 'open door' policy in general psychiatric hospitals has meant that offenders will not always be accepted and as there has been a reduction in the number of probation hostels, bail hostels are viewed as a necessary resource. Development of crisis intervention centres that provide or link into short-term accommodation is seen as a priority (NACRO, 1991b).

Similarly, in Birmingham a bail hostel is being set up to accommodate mentally disordered men. It is envisaged that referrals to this hostel will come from court teams, CPNs and bail information officers. The team is led by a nurse, and is to provide 24-hour care. It has initially been funded for 3 years to ascertain its cost effectiveness and will be constantly monitored and assessed (Thomas, 1993).

CPNs are seen as a crucial link between the criminal justice system and the health, social and voluntary services (Hillis, 1993; Chaloner and Kinsella, 1992).

There are several reasons why the CPN's role has been developed. CPNs are viewed as ambassadors for forensic psychiatry (Pederson, 1980) and they are seen as effective in liaising with agencies who normally work in isolation, and teaching and consultation are therefore important facets of the CPN's role (Chaloner and Kinsella, 1992). CPNs are less costly to employ than psychiatrists (Hedderman, 1993) and are thought to be more flexible because psychiatrists have other clinical commitments that cannot be cancelled at short notice (Cooke, 1992). Flexibility and responsiveness are seen as crucial to the effective working of these schemes; the psychiatrist can be brought in at a later stage if need be. James and Hamilton (1992) and Loo (1984) both indicate a need for a nursing assessment before allocating a hospital bed. Indeed, Loo (1984) suggested that a nurse's assessment would go some way to reassuring ward staff of the appropriateness of an 'offender' being placed in their care.

How do nurses work and what skills do they need?

Schemes for diverting the MDO vary greatly in their organizational styles. As a consequence, the CPN input into such schemes is equally diverse.

In order for a diversion scheme to function effectively, it requires a professional who can make skilled psychiatric assessments. The practicalities and difficulties of involving psychiatrists have already been described. However, it has been suggested that the involvement of the CPN offers a cost-effective alternative, because the CPN can carry out an 'initial screening'/ assessment.

The following are descriptive examples of different working models.

Panel schemes. In 1984 the Douglas Inch Centre was set up in Scotland as a treatment resource and alternative to custody for mentally disordered offenders (Cooke, 1992). However, it was in Hertfordshire, England that the first panel scheme was designed and operated in 1985. Mentally disordered offenders were mainly intercepted at the court stage of the criminal proceedings. This has since been extended to allow referral to the panel before the case comes to court and also when an MDO is expected to be discharged from a special hospital or prison. When a case is referred at court stage, the co-ordinator (probation officer) is informed by a referral form from the courts. The coordinator then convenes a panel, consisting of a CPN, psychologist and social worker, which agrees on the sentencing recommendations. These are put to the court via reports, such as a pre-sentence report. This 'management package', as it is called, is geared towards the needs of the individual and issues considered in it may include housing, education, social skills training, and so forth. If the police or Crown Prosecution Service (CPS) are concerned about a suspect's mental health they may contact the coordinator and/or CPN and ask for the suspect to be assessed for mental disorder. Once the panel's recommendations have been acted upon, the CPN becomes the case worker and liaises with the other professionals involved in supervising or caring for the client. The Hertfordshire panel scheme has not operated continuously since it began. It was initially developed by a group of professionals who were very committed but had little management support. Without a formalized structure and management support, the loss of one key individual resulted in the scheme faltering. Blumenthal and Wessely (1992) have found that this is a problem echoed in other areas. They describe such schemes as being initially dependent on the commitment and enthusiasm of individuals, and when these individuals leave there are often insufficient resources available to maintain a formalized approach to diversion schemes.

There is now diversion at the point of arrest, diversion at court, diversion of MDOs remanded in custody and the assessing and treating of mental health problems in prison. The Reaside Clinic, a regional secure unit (RSU) covering the West Midlands region and based in South Birmingham, has adopted all these approaches to divert MDOs and was initiated following the Circular 66/90 (Home Office, 1990; Hillis, 1993). Here, the CPN's role is seen as crucial to its implementation and effectiveness.

Diversion at the point of arrest. A pilot scheme has recently been set up at Bourneville Lane Police Station, Birmingham, to divert mentally disordered offenders at the point of arrest. Early data were referred to earlier. The nurse spent time at the station getting to know staff, understanding police procedures and devising complementary working practices. This was important to lay foundations for a successful partnership. The CPN is on call to interview anyone who is causing concern, prior to their being charged. Many who have been assessed by the CPN have been admitted to hospital. It is felt that the CPN is better able to assess a person for mental disorder than a police surgeon, who used to be the first person the custody officers contacted. Also, the CPNs have had more contacts within the health care system to bring about a more effective result (Cook, 1991). If the CPN is on site at the time the person is brought in, s/he observes the person through the booking process, with the intention of picking up information about, or indication of, the person's mental health. As a matter of course, people who are drunk or juveniles are not routinely interviewed.

If the CPN felt that the person had no mental health problems, the forensic medical examiner (FME) would not be called out. This has allowed for more constructive use of FMEs' time and for a more constructive disposal together with an increase in police confidence and awareness.

Diversion from court. The broad aims of the scheme include identifying people with mental disorder before their court appearance and offering advice to the CPS, Probation Service, police and others, to assist in making recommendations to the court. In addition, the aim is to arrange for people to be referred for assessment, treatment or admission to psychiatric hospitals when necessary, and to liaise with the court. Birmingham Magistrates' Courts consists of 24 separate courts (the largest court system in Europe). Defendants held in custody overnight from police stations throughout Birmingham are brought to a central 'lock-up' and are dealt with in one of these courts the next day. A CPN from Reaside Regional Secure Unit attends the central lock-up at 07.30 each morning, six days a week. S/he reads the CPS files on those detained, with the aim of identifying any defendants with potential mental health problems. The CPN has little time in which to identify which defendants need to be assessed, as the CPS must have the files back by 08.15. The criteria that the CPN uses to decide whether a defendant needs assessment are: those who have been charged with violent offences, e.g. murder, assault or wounding and sex offences; those charged on lesser offences whose behaviour has been described as bizarre or odd; and those with a known psychiatric history, who have made attempts at self-harm, or who may have a history of substance or alcohol abuse. Referrals are also made by police, solicitors and probation officers. Those identified are screened and their current mental health state is assessed, once the CPN has explained his/her role to the defendant, who can reject the assessment is s/he wishes; few people have refused (Hillis, 1993). The average number screened by one nurse is between two and six per day, between 08.30 and 09.30.

Assessments usually take place in the interview room, unless the defendant is considered to be disturbed, in which case s/he will be interviewed in the cell. The CPN has to take into consideration the possibility that the defendant may be very anxious before appearing in court and that s/he is being interviewed early in the morning.

After the initial screening, and before the court begins sitting at 10.00, discussions take place between the CPN, the CPS, the Bail Information Service and the liaison probation officer regarding those who have been identified as requiring intervention and diversion from custody.

The CPN's role is to persuade the CPS to discontinue the prosecution; this requires cooperation as CPNs cannot demand that a case be discontinued. The prosecution are less likely to discontinue the case, at this stage, if the charge is of a serious nature, essentially those involving violence (Cook, 1991).

If the CPN feels that the person should be assessed or treated as an outpatient, s/he contacts the relevant GP to make an appointment. Appropriate referral is also made for those suffering from substance or alcohol abuse. Referrals are only made with the defendant's consent. If it is apparent that the person needs admission to hospital, the court is requested to delay proceedings pending a full medical assessment by a psychiatrist.

Although CPNs are unable to make a full medical diagnosis, their in-depth assessments provide the court with an account of the presenting symptoms and contribute to the full medical assessment which is completed at a later stage. CPNs are responsible for making decisions about appropriate action, and will be influenced by the nature of the offence. A decision to discontinue proceedings can be considered only if the appropriate care has been arranged with the local services.

Placement in the RSU is considered for serious offences (such as murder or arson); discontinuance is not considered at this stage, but may occur later in the proceedings once the CPS has had adequate time to make that informed decision.

When compulsory admission is required under the Mental Health Act 1983, an approved social worker (ASW) is asked to attend. Reaside experienced some difficulty initially in obtaining an ASW when one was needed at short notice. They now have an ASW who assists in the liaison and provides support for the scheme. It also proved difficult to obtain medical support at short notice. To alleviate this problem, a senior registrar at Reaside (Section 12 approved under the Mental Health Act) agreed to provide the support required (Hillis, 1993). Compulsory admissions require two medical recommendations. They are usually made by either the catchment area psychiatrist, the police surgeon or the individual's GP. On completion of medical and ASW recommendations for hospital admission, the CPN then liaises with the CPS representative, who advises the court before the final decision is reached. The CPN then coordinates the admission with the ASW.

A CPN has been appointed to follow cases of MDOs who have been discontinued, bound over and conditionally discharged. This is to adopt a more proactive, rather than reactive, response to the needs of this client group. It is suggested that the support and follow-up given to these individuals may prevent re-offending. However, this suggestion will require empirical examination.

Support to remand prisoners. At Winson Green Prison, Birmingham, there is another pilot project involving a RMN. She visits all the newly remanded prisoners and screens them for evidence of potential self-harm, or a suicide risk, due to mental illness (Cohen, 1993). It is the first project of its kind in the country and, depending on its success, the Home Office may use this operational model in other jails across the country. The aim of the project is to facilitate the earliest possible identification of prisoners suffering mental health problems and to refer them to the most appropriate psychiatric service available. It may be possible to divert some from the prison system, depending on the seriousness of the charge. Compulsory admission to hospital and bail as a condition of continual treatment has already taken place as a direct result of this scheme being in operation.

After the screening process, the nurse reports any concerns about the prisoner's mental health to the health care officers in the prison. This may result in the inmate's transfer to an NHS resource, to the prisoner's hospital wing or to a period of close observation for up to 72 hours. If greater urgency is identified, the nurse will contact the GP to see the inmate immediately. The nurse emphasizes that it is of little value to have access only to a RMN to 'screen' prisoners: they also need to have contacts with other professionals such as probation officers and social worker, outside the prison, whom health care officers do not have access to (Cohen, 1993). The nurse attends court with the remanded inmate and emphasizes the need for diversion to hospital for treatment or community care. This is on the grounds that the inmate is vulnerable and could be a self-harm risk or be victimized by others (Cohen, 1993).

Initially the project was viewed as threatening by the health care officers in the prison. Such a shift in methods of working and perceived roles can cause stress in staff; the restrictiveness of the regime in secure environments can also lead to restrictiveness in staff attitudes to change (Neilson, 1992). Indeed, the health care officer may perceive the attention given to the inmate as manipulative (Reeder and Meldman, 1991). However, it is now seen as a valuable resource, particularly as the nurse has links with the 'outside' world and is able to use them rapidly to get to other forms of care. Winson Green prison has not had one suicide since the project began, and the number of self-harm incidents has dropped (Cohen, 1993).

A diversion scheme for mentally disordered offenders in Northampton was also set up as a result of the Circular 66/90. Northamptonshire has operated an adult reparation scheme for some considerable time (though not one orientated towards the needs of mentally disordered offenders) and the new scheme fits into this overall framework. A working group was formed to decide which disciplines should be involved in the diversion scheme. It identified a need for a probation officer, an approved social worker and a community-based psychiatric nurse.

Northampton's Diversion Unit (formerly Adult Reparation and Juvenile Liaison Bureau) duly consists of professionals from diverse backgrounds, e.g. police, teachers, social workers, probation and youth workers. Some members are permanent; some are seconded from their respective agencies. Currently, the CPNs are seconded for 2 years.

The need for a link with the health authority and for a professional experienced in dealing with mental disordered offenders influenced the decision to involve a nurse in the scheme. The disadvantage, however, is that most psychiatric nurses have little or no experience of or training in forensic psychiatry or of working with offenders and agencies in the criminal justice system. The local district health authorities (Northampton and Kettering) did not have a CPN with forensic experience in post and doubt was expressed that such work was within the remit of a generic CPN. The final recommendation was that a post should be set up specifically to meet this area.

The CPN acts as a specialist within the Diversion Unit, receiving referrals in his/her own right. In common with other schemes, s/he provides advice to the custody sergeants as to whether a person held in custody might be suffering from a mental disorder. What appears original to this scheme is the attention given to the victims. In addition to interviewing and assessing the offender, victims are also interviewed. If need be, the CPN will offer support to the victim or refer to an appropriate agency for this.

Referrals to the CPN can also be made at a number of other points in the process (Denton, 1993). Those MDOs who have committed a serious offence cannot be diverted from the criminal justice system but early contact with a CPN may facilitate later coordination between professionals such as a consultant psychiatrist preparing court reports and a probation officer preparing the pre-sentence report.

CONCLUSIONS

The aim of this study has been to review the CPN's role within diversion schemes. It was necessary to supplement the published material (as there was very little) with discussions with CPNs. An obvious feature of all schemes is that they provide for the assessment of those referred. It would be beneficial if they could all have a psychiatrist, as this might increase access to hospital beds when a need for admission has been identified. It has been indicated that a more cost-effective approach is to involve CPNs in carrying out initial screening assessments and for them then to make a judgement about the need for further assessment; not all mentally disordered offenders require in-depth psychiatric assessment. Also, if the outcome of the assessment is a recommendation that the offender needs care in the community, then the CPN's combination of skills in liaison, links between different systems (criminal justice, health and social services) and understanding of the needs of the client group make them the best placed individuals to take on the role of supervising the offender or make decisions about onward referral (Pearse, 1993).

There is a need to develop training in this area of work (Reed, 1992). One aspect of this training should be in multi-agency working with mentally disordered offenders, particularly in the light of the criticism in the Clunis report (Home Office, 1994) of the lack of multi-agency facilities. There is also a need to develop specialist training for CPNs, perhaps under the auspices of the English National Board, or other concerned organizations.

The role of the CPN in diverting mentally disordered offenders is still being developed. However, even at this early stage, it is possible to identify some of the core skills required by nurses working in this setting. Hillis (1993) views CPNs as having a pivotal role, both between the client and the various agencies and between the various agencies themselves. Skills in liaison are crucial: the CPN is involved in working with a diversity of systems. It is important that the CPN achieves credibility with agencies who traditionally view 'caring professionals' with suspicion. The work carried out in Birmingham, at Bourneville Lane Police Station and at Winson Green Prison, demonstrate that such credibility can be achieved.

Psychiatric nursing has had little in the way of its own ideology upon which to base its practice. Thus, nurses have taken on the ideologies and assumptions of other dominant professions, notably psychiatry (Adams, 1990). Adams noted the development of a trend towards democracy in community mental health teams and a 'devolution' of the traditional hierarchy. This trend has led to an increasing autonomy in community psychiatric nursing practice. This will certainly be true of CPNs working in diversion schemes, where the separation from psychiatry is all the greater, the CPN often being the only health professional in a diversion team. While this may help psychiatric nursing as a whole develop its own ideology and identity, it is not without potential problems. Nurses may find themselves being managed by professionals who do not have an awareness of (say) the obligations of the UKCC Code of Conduct (UKCC, 1992). Issues such as confidentiality, for example, can be understood differently by different professionals. This is a potential source of conflict. Another important issue is that of clinical supervision. A non-nursing supervisor may have an understanding of the issues concerning mentally disordered offenders but not of those specific to nurses. The converse may be true if a nurse supervisor is chosen, since nurses with adequate experience in this field are likely to remain in short supply for quite some time.

It is clear from the demands that this particular client group make that CPNs in diversion schemes should have smaller caseloads than would normally be expected in generic community psychiatric nursing. This is especially important if CPNs are to maintain the responsiveness that has been characteristic of their role in the schemes described.

Advocacy has been identified as an important part of the CPN's role. Higgins (1991) writes of need to 'sell' such clients to other agencies and identifies issues such as housing where this has always proved difficult.

It is again clear from the work completed in Birmingham that considerable skills in assessment are required, with possibly several assessments having to be carried out in a very short period of time.

The CPN needs to be sensitive to issues of illness, personality and social factors, all of which may have contributed to the offence. In addition to assessment, CPNs will need to have a broad range of therapeutic skills and to be aware of the therapeutic issues for offenders and for victims if Northamptonshire's model is to be more widely adopted. Higgins (1991) comments that the use of these staff cannot be undervalued as their caseload is remarkable.

It has been established that diverting is the more humane answer to dealing with MDOs. It has been suggested that diversion schemes can reduce both costs and recividism. As yet there is no evidence to support this, and it is a widely held belief that community care is substantially more expensive than institutional care.

In developing diversion schemes there is a need for sensitivity to issues of public concern and safety, particularly in light of the recent Clunis report (Home Office, 1994). Similarly, there is the issue of whether an offender may want to be labelled 'mentally disordered' and be subsequently diverted from the criminal justice system or whether s/he wants the opportunity to be found not guilty of the offence within the court system.

The present study found a paucity of literature available regarding diversion schemes. There were published data regarding the historical context for the inception of diversion schemes, but less on the evaluation of their effectiveness (diversion schemes are still relatively new) and very little on the CPN's role within diversion schemes. This study has therefore necessarily been limited. However, as new services are developed, it is to be expected that rigorous evaluations will follow and eventually enter the public domain for critical review.

ACKNOWLEDGEMENTS

Thanks are due to Dorothy Tonak for her help in the writing of this chapter.

REFERENCES

Adams, T. (1990) A model of multidisciplinary team working. *Senior Nurse*, **10**, 13–16.
Barnum, P. (1992) *Closing the Asylum*, Penguin, Harmondsworth.

Black, T. (1984) Treatment in maximum security settings, in *Mentally Abnormal Offender*, (eds M. Craft and A. Craft), Baillière Tindall, Eastbourne, p. 350–83.

Bluglass, R. (1993) Introduction, in *Implementing Interagency Initiatives for Mentally Disordered Offenders*, (eds D. Tonak and H. Rees), p. 22–5 Tonak, Buckingham.

Blumenthal, S. and Wessely, S. (1992) National survey of current arrangements for diversion from custody in England and Wales. *British Medical Journal*, **305**, 1322–5.

Burrows, S. (1993) Inside the walls. *Nursing Times*, **89**, 38–40.

Butler Report (1975) *Report of the Committee on Mentally Abnormal Offenders*, Cmnd 6244, HMSO, London.

Chaloner, C. and Kinsella, C. (1992) Care with conviction. *Nursing Times*, **88**, 50–2.

Cheswick, D. (1992) Reed report on mentally disordered offenders: they need health and social services not prison. *British Medical Journal*, **305**, 1448–9.

Cohen, P. (1993) Remanded in safe custody. *Nursing Times*, **89**, 14–15.

Coids, J. (1988) Mentally abnormal offenders on remand. *British Medical Journal*, **296**, 1779–82

Cook, I. (1991) Springing the trap. *Nursing Times*, **87**, 16–17.

Cooke, D.I. (1992) Reconviction following referral to a forensic clinic: the criminal outcome of diversion. *Medicine, Science and the Law*, **32**, 325–30.

Courtney, P. and Cunnane, J. (1992) provision of secure psychiatric services in Leeds; Paper 2. A survey of unmet needs. *Health Trends*, **24**.

Dell, S. and Robertson, G. (1993) Remands and psychiatric assessment in Holloway prison: the psychotic population. *British Journal of Psychiatry*, **163**, 634–6.

Denton, P. (1993) Diversion unit referral process when there is concern regarding mental state. Unpublished material from Northamptonshire's Division Unit.

Department of Health (1992) *The Health of the Nation*. HMSO, London.

Dietz, P. (1992) Mentally disordered offenders. Patterns in the relationship between mental disorder and crime. *Clinical Forensic Psychiatry*, **15**, 539–51.

Dobson, G. (1992) Papers from participating services, in *Implementing Interagency Initiatives for Mentally Disordered Offenders*, (eds. D. Tonak and H. Rees), Tonak, Buckingham, p. 41–4.

Everall, D. (1993) 'CHIPS': a resource for mentally disordered offenders. Community health integrated programme services, in *Implementing Interagency Initiatives for the Mentally Disordered Offenders*, (eds. D. Tonak and H. Rees), Tonak, Buckingham, p. 160.

Freeman, R. and Roesch, R. (1989) Mental disorder and the criminal justice system: a review. Special issue: Mental disorder and the criminal justice system. *International Journal of Law and Psychiatry*, **12**, 105–15.

Glancy, J.E. (1974) *Report of the Working Party on NHS Psychiatric Hospitals*, HMSO, London.

Gostin, L. (1984) Towards the development of principles for sentencing and detaining mentally abnormal offenders, in *Mentally Abnormal Offender*, (eds M. Craft and A. Craft), Baillière Tindall, Eastbourne, p. 224–41.

Griffiths, D. (1993) Newsletter, National Practitioners Group, Mentally Disordered Offenders, 2nd edn, West Midlands.

Gunn, J. (1979) The law and the mentally abnormal offender, in England and Wales. *International Journal of Law and Psychiatry*, **2**, 199–214.

176 *Community psychiatric nurses and diversion schemes*

Gunn, J. (1981) Questions and reponsibility and the Sutcliffe case. *Poly Law Review*, 66–70

Gunn, J. (1991) *The Number of Psychiatric Cases amongst Sentenced Prisoners*. HMSO, London.

Hedderman, C. (1993) *Panel Assessment Schemes for Mentally Disordered Offenders* Research and Planning Unit, Home Office, paper 76, HMSO, London.

Higgins, J. (1991) The mentally disordered offender in the community, in *Mentally Disordered Offenders* (eds K. Herbs and J. Gunn), Butterworth-Heinemann, London, p. 171–85.

Hillis, G. (1993) Diverting tactics. *Nursing Times*, **89** 24–27.

Hoggett, B. (1990) *Mental Health Law*, 3rd edn. Sweet & Maxwell, London.

Home Office (1990) *Provision for Mentally Disordered Offenders*, Circular 66/90, HMSO, London.

Home Office (1994) *The Report of the Inquiry into the Care and Treatment of Christopher Clunis*, North East Thames and South East Thames Regional Health Authority, HMSO, London.

James, D.V. and Hamilton, L.W. (1991) The Clerkenwell scheme: assessing the efficacy and cost of a psychiatric liaison service to a magistrates court. *British Medical Journal*, **303**, 285.

James, D.V. and Hamilton, L.W. (1992) Setting up psychiatric liaison schemes to magistrate courts: problems and practicalities. *Medicine, Science and Law*, **32**, 167–76.

Johnson, C. and Smith, J. (1993) What else can we do? New initiatives in diversion from custody. *Justice of the Peace*, **157**, 280–1.

Jones, D. and Dean, N. (1992) Assessment of needs for services for mentally disordered with patients with similar needs. *Health Trends*, **24**, 48.

Joseph, P. (1992) *Psychiatric Assessment at the Magistrates' Court*, Report Commissioned by the Home Office, HMSO, London.

Lawson, W.K. (1984) Mentally abnormal offenders in prisons in *Mentally Abnormal Offender*, (eds M. Craft and A. Craft), Baillière Tindall, Eastbourne, p.154–76.

Loo, A. (1984) A secure provision. *Nursing Times*, **2 May**, 44–6.

McMillan, I. (1993) Widening the safety net. *Nursing Times*, 89.

Morrison, E.F. (1991) Victimization in prison: implications for the mentally ill inmate and for health professionals. *Archives of Psychiatric Nursing*, **5**, 17–24.

Mustill, M. (1991) Some concluding reflections, in *Mentally Disordered Offenders* (eds K. Herbs and J. Gunn), Butterworth-Heinemann, London, p. 225–47.

NACRO (1991a) Policy Paper 2: *Diverting Mentally Disturbed Offenders from Prosecution*. NACRO, London.

NACRO (1991b) Policy Paper 1: *Community Care and Mentally Disturbed Offenders*. NACRO, London.

Neilson, P. (1992) A secure provision. *Nursing Times*, **88**, 31–3.

Pearse, R. (1993) Newsletter, 2nd edn, National Practitioners Group, Mentally Disordered Offenders, West Midlands.

Pederson, P. (1980) The role of community psychiatric nurses in forensic psychiatry. *Community Psychiatric Nursing Journal*, **8**, 12–17.

Percy Commission (1957) *Roual Commission on the Law relating to Mental Illness and Mental Deficiency*, 1954–7, Cmnd 169, HMSO, London.

Pitt, R. (1993) Who cares? *Nursing Times*, **89**, 27–9.

Reed, J. (1992) *Review of Health and Social Services for Mentally Disordered Offenders and Others Requiring Similar Services: Final Summary Report*, Cmnd 2088, HMSO, London.

Reeder, D. and Meldman, L. (1991) Conceptualising psycho-social nursing in the jail setting. *Journal of Psychosocial Nursing and Mental Health Services*, **29**, 40–1; 46–7.

Rice, M.E. and Harris, G.T. (1992) A comparison of criminal recidivism among schizophrenic and non-schizophrenic offenders. *International Journal of Law and Psychiatry*, **15**, 397–408.

Robertson, G. (1988) Arrest patterns among mentally disordered offenders. *British Journal of Psychiatry*, **153**, 313–16.

Sadler, C. (1989) Held without help. *Nursing Times*, **84**, 16–17.

Shaw, S. and Simpson, A. (1991) Thro' cells of madness: the imprisonment of mentally ill people, in *Mentally Disordered Offenders*, (eds K. Herbs and J. Gunn), Butterworth-Heinemann, London, p. 104–16.

Spurgeon, D. (1993) Newsletter, 2nd edn, National Practitioners Group. Mentally Disordered Offenders, West Midlands.

Staite, C. and Martin, N. (1993) What else can we do? New initiatives in diversion from custody. *Justice of the Peace*, **157**, 280–1.

Stuart-White, C. (1991) The 'inadequate' offender: a view from the courts, in *Mentally Disordered Offenders*, (eds K. Herbs and J. Gunn), Butterworth-Heinemann, London, p. 65–79.

Thomas, L. (1993) Newsletter, 2nd edn, National Practitioners Group, Mentally Disordered Offenders, West Midlands.

UKCC (1992) *Code of Professional Conduct*, United Kingdom Central Council for Nursing, Midwifery and Health Visiting, London.

Walker, N. and McCabe, S. (1973) *Crime and Insanity in England 2: New Solutions and New Problems*, Edinburgh University Press, Edinburgh.

West, D.J. and Walker, A. (1977) *Daniel McNaughton: His Trial and the Aftermath*, Gaskell Books, London.

Woolfe, H. and Tumin, S. (1990) *Prison Disturbances: The Report of an Enquiry*, (The Woolfe Report), HMSO, London.

CHAPTER TEN

Mental health nursing and case management

Richard Ford

INTRODUCTION

In 1955 inpatient services dominated specialist mental health care with a peak of 150 000 beds (Davidge *et al.*, 1993) and nursing care was correspondingly hospital-based. At this time community psychiatric nursing services were first established and by 1990 White (1990) estimated that there were nearly 5000 community psychiatric nurses (CPNs). During this period hospital inpatient beds had fallen dramatically to under 60 000 (Davidge *et al.*, 1993). In addition to the continued growth in the number of CPNs, mental health nurses now work in specialist community teams and as case (or care) managers. Furthermore, mental health nurses work in various forms of residential care and day care. The last 40 years have therefore seen a fundamental change both in the settings in which mental health nursing takes place and in the diversity of ways in which it is practised.

While the late 1980s saw considerable de-institutionalization it was not until the early 1990s that there was extensive legislation and policy guidance. More recently the development of the legislative framework has been prompted by a rising tide of critical public opinion over perceived failings of community care. The policy response in the UK has, as in the US, had forms of case management at its core. Case management places considerable emphasis on making contact through assertive outreach, followed by comprehensive assessment of client need, developing a negotiated package of care, direct care provision, care coordination, monitoring and review (Ryan, Ford and Clifford, 1991). Both the Care Programme Approach (CPA) (DoH, 1990), with the appointment of keyworkers, and care management (DoH, 1991) have their roots in case management. Care management tends to emphasize direct work with clients. Neither care management or keyworking necessarily employs assertive outreach to link clients with services and to maintain long-term contact.

The Research and Development for Psychiatry/Department of Health Case Management Project was established in 1989 and went on to provide a service to over 700 clients (Ford *et al.*, 1993a) in six localities. This development preceded both the CPA and care management. While the White Paper *Caring for People* (DoH, 1989) referred to 'case' management, subsequent guidance (DoH, 1991) has changed the term to 'care' management. Care management refers specifically, in the UK context, to local authority purchasing of social care through assessment, care planning, coordinating and monitoring. To avoid confusion the original, and more generic, term of 'case management' is used in this chapter. All the services focused on assertive outreach and the development of a long-term supportive relationship with clients. Case managers undertook considerable direct work with their clients, although they did not use any specific therapeutic interventions. Care coordination and advocacy were highlighted but formal purchasing was not undertaken. Case managers worked Monday to Friday 9 a.m.–5 p.m. with limited ability to work more flexibly, without any attempt to provide a 24-hour service. Teams were recruited from a variety of professional backgrounds but undertook generic work with direct management from their team leader, irrespective of profession. Forging strong links with psychiatrists was emphasized by all the teams. The role of the psychiatrist varied from that of clinical director through specialist consultancy for the team to individual client-based input. Equally important was liaison and cooperation between case managers and general practitioners.

As community care continues to develop, with plans for closure of all but 30 of the 'water tower hospitals' by the end of the century (Davidge *et al.*, 1993), the diversification of nursing will continue and will be heavily influenced by policy developments dominated by case management approaches. Many nurses will indeed see considerable similarity between case management and modern mental health nursing, which seeks to plan care within a holistic approach. This chapter seeks to clarify the differences between these approaches and discuss the implications for mental health nurses.

METHOD

Wooff, Goldberg and Fryers (1988) used observational methods to delineate differences between CPNs and social workers. However, this method was not feasible for this study as the considerable researcher time needed was not available. Another method that enabled a detailed description of how CPNs

1.2.2   What criteria are used for selecting clients to work with?

        PROMPT: are any particular groups targeted?

Please answer all further questions with the long term client group in mind

2.2.2   Do you have clients who you feel should probably stay on your caseload indefinitely?

2.3.1   What do you do if a client is usually out or says they don't want to see you?

2.4.2   Are there any tasks/activities that need doing in relation to this client group that you do not consider appropriate for you to do?

        PROMPT: Injection giving

              Helping with household tasks

              Taking client to a social activity

              Helping with a benefit claim

              Assessing effects of medication

              Monitoring symptoms

              Physical health-related tasks (e.g. bathing)

2.5.1   In your view, what are the similarities and differences between the role of the CM and the role of the CPN?

2.6.1   What do you feel you achieve for the client in your work?

        PROMPT: i.e. what is the outcome of your work, not what you hope to do

        Selected individual client

3.1   Who has responsibility for the client?

3.2   What are your overall goals?

3.6   Would you like to put more time into your work with this client?

3.7   Could you put too much time in?

3.8   Please can you describe the type of care that you have been giving to this client over the last 6 months.

Figure 10.1 Case manager and community psychiatric nurse interview (developed by Richard Ford; copyright ©. Research and Development for Psychiatry 1992).

make community psychiatric nursing work was the repertory grid as used by Pollock (1988). The data collected proved difficult to quantify (Pollock, 1990) and would not allow for ready comparison between groups. Tyrer *et al.* (1990) used a highly standardized method to investigate the relationship between client diagnosis and specific interventions. Such an approach, while providing quantitative data, does not allow for discovery of the nature of interventions. Our earlier research work within the Case Management Project (Ford *et al.*, 1993b; Repper, Ford and Cooke, 1994) and the work of Barratt (1989) suggested that semi-structured interviews with CMs and CPNs would be both feasible, quantifiable at a descriptive level and discover the nature of the work undertaken by the two groups. This earlier work and a review of previous studies of community psychiatric nursing informed the interview guide in Figure 10.1 (only questions used for material presented here are reproduced).

As there were many CMs who had practised as nurses there was an ideal opportunity to look at the work of CMs and CPNs from the perspective of people who had carried out both roles. For the sub-study reported here 10 CPNs, 10 CMs from a nursing background and 10 CMs from a non-nursing background were interviewed using a semi-structured guide. The sample of CMs and CPNs were recruited on the four main research sites of the project. Respondents were selected on the basis of their availability whilst attempting to match on the characteristics shown in Table 10.1.

Table 10.1 Case manager and community psychiatric nurse characteristics (CM(N) = Case manager with nursing qualification; CM(non) = Case manager without nursing qualification; CPN = Community psychiatric nurse)

	CM(N) (n = 10)	CM(non) (n = 10)	CPN (n = 10)
Male	5	6	4
Age 40 or under	6	8	5
Educated to A level or above	7	7	4
Educated to degree level	3	6	1
10 years or more experience	7	5	8
10 years or more with long-term clients	3	1	6
Additional formally asssessed training	6	5	9
Mean caseload size	10	15	54

All nurses in the sub-study held a first level qualification except two of the former nurses who had become CMs. Eight of the CMs who were not former nurses held social work qualifications. The three groups were broadly similar in their characteristics except that the CMs without nursing qualifications tended to be younger, less experienced and more likely to be educated to degree level, but had undertaken less post-qualification training. Mean caseload size varied considerably. Although all respondents had a majority of clients with severe and persistent mental health problems, for CMs this was their exclusive client group. This chapter explores case management and community psychiatric nursing; it does not attempt to investigate the influence of having a nursing background for CMs.

Interviews were carried out by the author (RF) and lasted an average of 1 hour. All interviews were audiotaped and transcribed. Interviewee responses were studied and coding frameworks developed for each question. This analysis allowed the responses to be structured and for descriptive statistics to be produced. Typical instances of responses are given here which allow the reader to more fully understand the work of case managers and CPNs as portrayed by them.

FINDINGS

Similarities and differences

Many CMs and CPNs felt that most of their work was similar (Table 10.2). However, they did not go on to detail the nature of the similarities between their roles, rather, they sought to relate the differences they perceived. The differences described by CMs and CPNs (Q2.5.1 and Q2.5.2) were predicted in the interview design and are therefore all covered by separate specific questions. Some of these specific questions may have prompted responses to these general questions, although there is some evidence that this was not the case. For example, the question covering the most frequently mentioned difference, the greater time that CMs had for their work (Q3.6), was asked after the question on similarities and differences.

Table 10.2 Ways in which the CM role differs from that of the CPN

Areas mainly identified by CMs
- CM covers all areas – no boundaries to the role
- CMs do more care coordination
- CMs focus on serious mental health problems
- CMs client-centred
- CM involves assertive outreach/engagement
- CMs have responsibility

Areas mainly identified by CPNs
- CMs create dependency
- CMs only have a social care role
- Don't know about the CM role

Areas identified by CMs and CPNs
- CM and CPN roles similar in most respects
- CMs have the time
- CMs have a longer-term role

Open questions of this type generate varying lengths of response from interviewees and CPNs identified fewer differences in roles than did CMs. This was probably because of CMs' greater familiarity with both roles.

For this reason comparisons between CMs' and CPNs' responses to these questions need to be made with caution. Yet there are some general observations that can be made. All three groups of interviewees felt that CMs had more time than CPNs for their work. While CMs felt their work to be broader and more holistic, to involve more coordination, to be more client-centred and to involve more assertive outreach, few CPNs saw these differences. Indeed half the CPNs interviewed felt that one of the differences was that CMs made their clients dependent on them, a view not shared by the CMs.

The main advantage of these open questions was to generate themes for further exploration. In this way the expressed differences in roles between CMs and CPNs given in response to this question provides a useful framework for the discussion of the other findings of this sub-study.

Having the time

The extra time available to CMs, as a result of smaller caseloads, was the most prevalent response from all three groups (Q2.5.1) but when asked specifically (Q3.6) if they would like to have more time to put into their work, only two CPNs said that they would (similarly two people in each case-manager group also wanted more time). This apparently contradictory finding can be explained. CPNs have developed their role to fit in with the demands of having high caseloads. If they had more time there would be little benefit from providing more of the same type of care; they would have to develop an expanded or extended role. However, when they do not have the increased time they do not think hypothetically about what they would do with it. Therefore, the response that CMs have more time, which enables CMs to fulfil a different role, is congruent with the response that they do not need more time to fulfil their own roles as CPNs. These responses suggest that, while the CM role is dependent on having more time, it is not an expansion of the CPN role, rather it is a different role.

Focus on specific client group

CMs had a remit to work with a very specific client group. All but one CM were able to list the criteria for accepting or rejecting clients (Q1.2.2). The criteria for acceptance included people with a psychotic diagnosis, with multiple needs, where there were difficulties in coordinating the care inputs of several agencies, especially where the client had difficulty accessing or accepting care. In comparison the opposite was true for CPNs, with only one CPN responding that there were any criteria at all for who they worked with.

Table 10.3 Number of respondents reporting each category of desired length of client contact

	CM(N) (n = 10)	CM(non) (n = 10)	CPN (n = 10)
Indefinite contact	9	2	4
Negotiable with client and other services	1	8	0
Short-term contact	0	0	6

CMs were also more likely to say that they would keep clients on their caseload indefinitely or that this was negotiable (Table 10.3, Q2.2.2). CPNs were more likely to want to see some throughput on their caseload.

Taking responsibility

There has been mounting public concern that people with severe mental health problems are not receiving adequate community care. As a result the Health Secretary has announced a 10-point plan for developing successful and safe community care (DoH, 1993). The first point of her plan is a proposal to amend the Mental Health Act 1984 to allow for 'Supervised Discharge'. This increases the responsibility of community-based mental health nurses already working within the existing aftercare provisions of Section 117 of the Act and the Care Programme Approach (DoH, 1990).

When asked 'who is responsible for the client?' (Q3.1) CMs were usually clear that they took overall responsibility and that, in contrast to CPNs, this was not shared among a team of professionals (Table 10.4). A CM felt that it was her responsibility to maintain contact with vulnerable clients. She found it stressful when someone was actively refusing a service, but was reassured when she felt some form of contact was being maintained: 'It is our responsibility to go out and search for them, to make sure they are alright. That means calling and calling and leaving notes. There is the odd case when they are there. So there is persistent contact and also it is reassuring to me that they are alright.'

Table 10.4 Number of respondents reporting each category of responsibility for care provision

	CM(N) (n = 10)	CM(non) (n = 10)	CPN (n = 10)
Sole responsibility	4	8	2
Shared responsibility	2	1	6
Others responsible	4	1	2

Assertive engagement

In the current environment of increased responsibility, when clients who are assessed to be in need of services do not find these acceptable, mental health workers will not be able to give up, or merely pass them back to referrers. It is imperative that mental health workers find a way of working with these clients.

How then can the link between clients and appropriate mental health services be made? Following the successful work of Stein and Test (1982) in the US an approach that has become popular in many countries is 'assertive outreach'. Stein and Test describe this vividly: 'If someone does not show up for an appointment . . . we will go out and find the person. . . . When we find the person we don't hit him (or her) over the head, shanghai him, and haul him back into the program; but we do stop him, talk to him, and try to convince him that we would really like to get reinvolved with him.'

After 12–18 months of case management 94% of clients accepted for the service were in contact with appropriate services (Ford, Cooke and Repper, 1992; Ford *et al.*, 1994a). After 3 years of the study this figure has increased to 96% based on the follow-up of 330 clients (Ford *et al.*, 1994b). These figures were significantly higher than those for a randomly selected control group ($n = 38$) where 28% fell out of care.

In this sub-study 90% (18 out of 20) of CMs said they would continue indefinitely trying to build a relationship with the client, compared to only 10% (one out of 10) of CPNs (Q2.3.1). This result was expected as CPNs had three times as many clients on their books and talked of having to give up quickly so as to make space for new referrals. No CPN said they would accept a client's refusal to see them on the first occasion, but all would have passed the case back to the referrer, usually the GP, within six attempts.

CMs carrying out assertive outreach persisted indefinitely, whatever the circumstances. As a CM said: 'there is only so much you can take, running down the road with someone chasing you with a half brick, which has happened, but I have stuck with it. I mean, that particular person, I stuck with that for 9 months. Now I'm the best thing since sliced bread.' By persisting this CM now has a long-term supportive relationship with the client and an appropriate package of care is being delivered.

CMs developed a 'rule of thumb' to help them assess the need to provide assertive outreach: 'If we think the person is telling us to leave because they are overtly ill we don't pay as much attention to it. If they are coping well enough and their judgement is not too impaired we accept that.'

Inevitably, this 'rule of thumb' judgement was difficult to make and case managers would opt for keeping arms length contact so that they could regularly monitor the situation. 'I will ring around and try and find what the person's routine is. If they have a circle of friends I will contact them. If they don't want to see me that's fine, but I will try and keep an eye, to try and monitor the client, by seeking other people's opinions.'

This CM went on to say that if he had any concerns he would not discharge the person as they were in need of help.

In their attempts to build long-term relationships CMs would try and discuss or negotiate their contact with the client: 'Early on people will say they don't want a service. We try to negotiate so the person can give us a bit of time. We can get to know them better. They can understand a bit more about what our service has to offer.'

This CM was happy to negotiate as it had the additional benefit of allowing enough time for some rapport to develop. There were many examples where case managers preferred this strategy to direct confrontation. They also recognized that there was an element of risk-taking attached as they did not have ideal contact.

CMs were prepared to accept that they may only be able to have a limited involvement with the client, yet this was seen as far preferable to no involvement. In these circumstances CMs were not able to be proactive in their work but they could react to any deterioration in their client's circumstances. For example, a client might eventually need to be admitted. During the subsequent treatment period case managers were able to work intensively to build their relationship with the client. This was a useful basis for more effective maintenance in the community following discharge. One CM described the way that she worked constructively with the client whilst she was in hospital: 'while she was in hospital we managed to talk about what she wanted most and then I moved from her first priority being never to see me again. That moved to priority number three. Priorities one and two became things that involved seeing me, so she would agree to see me until those things were done.' Many CMs talked about working in this client-centred way, which is further investigated below (page 189).

An assertive outreach approach has been demonstrated as being effective in maintaining contact with clients. Within a case management framework this involved considerable persistence on the part of the CM. There were also difficult judgements to be made between exercising responsibility for the needs of vulnerable clients and the right of clients to refuse services. To help make these decisions, and to dissipate the stress involved in assertive outreach, high-quality clinical supervision is needed.

Doing anything

Having established that case management is not just about having more time to do the same thing, what is it that CMs and CPNs actually do? A total of 95% (19 out of 20) of CMs reported that they would undertake a wide variety of tasks as a regular part of their role compared to 20% (two out of 10) CPNs (Q2.4.2). The other eight CPNs said that they would occasionally take on these tasks but did not see them as part of their role. CPNs reported in general

Table 10.5 Types of work undertaken by CMs and CPNs

Areas identified mainly by CMs
- Housing and finance
- Daily living skills
- Interpersonal relationships
- Social contact
- Legal

Areas identified mainly by CPNs
- Medication
- Specific psychosocial interventions

Areas identified by CMs and CPNs
- Relatives/carers support
- Non-specific support for the client
- Monitoring mental state
- Client employment

---

that they had to do these things on occasions as they could see the client suffer, but these were tasks that they felt they should not have to do.

When asked about the specific care that they had given to an individual client the responses showed that CMs were more involved in the areas of housing/finance, interpersonal relationships, social contact, daily living skills and legal matters (Table 10.5) (Q3.8). Some of the examples given by CMs show both the broad range of areas they were involved with and the lengths they would go to provide care. For instance the following case study described (précis retaining the CM's own words) by a CM covered all the areas of Table 10.5, yet was not atypical of CMs' responses:

The major problem was to get him to hospital as his condition had deteriorated. But, he didn't see the need. So I sought medical opinion and he was admitted under section 2. For about 6 weeks he was on the ward and I was in twice a week liaising with the ward staff and assisting with the ward programme. Then I was implementing the section 117 aftercare programme, which was attending occupational therapy three times a week and a weekly review with the consultant – and making sure he does attend.

His flat was in a state, he had no electricity or gas for a long time. First, while he was in hospital I got the flat fumigated, the rubbish cleared and the electricity rewired and the gas recommissioned. I went to the Salvation Army place and they gave us a truckful of furniture for his place, some carpets, cooking pots and clothes.

He was discharged to his parents' home. So I assisted him and his father to clean the kitchen, the living room and to lay the carpets in his flat.

We've done that now. I arranged for a community care grant for him. He was given £700, but now it's to hand he doesn't want to spend it! He had a fire in his place and I don't think his gas cooker is safe but he is insisting that it is safe and that it only needs cleaning. So, I am negotiating with him that we get rid of that one and buy a cheap secondhand one.

There is a problem with his neighbours because he was disturbed prior to when he went into hospital. He used to shout and his behaviour was generally very very upsetting towards them. I have regular meetings with the Estates Officer and the tenants reps to reassure them that his behaviour was due to the fact that he wasn't well and he is being treated and he is now staying with his parents and by the time he returns he should be OK.

In comparison CPNs were more likely to report that their care related to medication and forms of specific psychotherapeutic interventions, such as bereavement counselling or social skills training. CPNs also tended to cover fewer areas in less depth. The following example was the most comprehensive description (précis) of care provided by a CPN:

I have been giving regular injections once a month and monitoring his mental state. I have taken him to day centres, I have referred him on to the employment officer. We have done a bit of role play with how to get into a garage and get your car MOT. Lots of support and social things with mum. Like chatting and if she's got worries we discuss those. I'm alone with the client some of the time and then he will discuss what he has been doing and how much exercise he's been taking. He's got on to the exercise machine which is quite good. This lad's amazing, I'm telling you, he didn't do anything for 12 months, a little bit of antidepressant medication, quite an improvement, he's ready now to move on to a flat. A lot of the work has to be done with mum letting go of him.

Of course the two case studies provided here cannot be directly compared. The CM visited the client six times a month, compared to the CPN's two. By having low caseloads, and consequently the time, the flexibility of the case management approach allows the CM to undertake a broader array of tasks, at a greater depth.

Both groups talked about their work with relatives, offering non-specific support, the general monitoring of their clients' mental state and work. Other areas that were mentioned by two or less people in any group were physical health care and education.

By focusing on social care as opposed to treatment CMs were able to engage clients with services. Usually clients wanted help with practical matters such as accommodation and finance. They were seldom interested in medication in its own right. As clients were motivated to deal with practical matters these were considered first. Often it was possible to increase clients' motivation to deal with medication issues when these could be linked to the practical interests of the client. For example medication could be seen as enabling a client to pursue some kind of occupation.

Arranging care

When CMs and CPNs were asked about their work with one specific client (Q3.8) all groups reported high levels of care coordination activitiy (Table 10.6). Closer analysis revealed that while both CMs and CPNs undertook considerable general liaison work for the majority of their clients, CMs were involved in arranging additional care for their clients. To succssfully arrange care they described how they actively advocated on behalf of their clients and how they then undertook to go with their clients to the new care settings to ensure that engagement occurred.

Table 10.6 Types of care coordination undertaken by CMs and CPNs

Areas identified mainly by CMs
- Arranging care
- Advocacy
- Engaging client with other agencies

Areas identified mainly by CPNs
- General liaison

Areas identified by CMs and CPNs
- Care coordination in general

A CPN, for example, discussed how she liaised with ward staff, day centre staff, home help, bathing service, meals-on-wheels and a trainee GP for one client with multiple disabilities. While this CPN liaised with all these people she made it clear that the client's daughter was responsible for organizing care and that she, as a CPN, was only responsible for her own care input. In somewhat similar circumstances a CM detailed the agencies that he had contact with: sheltered accommodation wardens, several medical out-patient clinics, psychiatric out-patient clinic and home help. In contrast to the CPN, the CM sees his main function as being a coordinator. He went with the client to her appointments, monitored the inputs of other agencies through regular contacts and 'coordinated their inputs into discussion reviews'.

Achieving what the client wants

The work of Rapp (1993) had a considerable influence on the RDP Case Management Project. This approach places emphasis on clients directing the aims of their own care and concentrates on building upon their strengths, rather than focusing on their disabilities. Rapp's 'strengths' approach was most vident in CMs' responses, in particular responses from non-nurses, when asked about their achievements for clients in general (Table 10.7, Q2.6.1).

Table 10.7 Types of achievement aimed for by CMs and CPNs

Areas identified mainly by CMs
- 'What the client wants'
- Housing/welfare

Areas identified mainly by CPNs
- Prevention of relapse
- Medication compliance
- Independence
- Improved confidence
- Internal growth

Areas identified by CMs and CPNs
- Improved quality of life in general
- Empathic relationship between client and worker
- Client engagement with care
- Low expectations of achievement

However, when asked about their goals for individual clients (Q3.2) only five CMs mentioned anything connected to the expressed desires of the client. Furthermore, when asked about the care that they delivered (Q3.8), no CMs said that they did what the client wanted on a day-to-day basis. At the time of interviewing, the influence of the strengths approach appears to have been at a more overall, philosophical level than at a day-to-day practice level. This client-led orientation was emphasized by one CM in the following style (Q2.6): 'Well, I hope that whatever they want to achieve is, within reason, achievable. That is probably a better life style. I suppose that covers your living environment, your social, financial – whatever it takes really.' CMs also felt they achieved improved housing and welfare benefits for their clients which corresponds to the actual work they undertook (Table 10.5). Coupled with their client-led philosophical orientation this suggests that the case management approach did not have any specific professional demarcation; indeed the client-centredness of the approach militates against the recognition of any boundaries.

In comparison CPNs felt that they prevented relapse and consequent readmission to hospital, and improved medication compliance. Also CPNs were more likely to feel that they achieved psychological and psychosocial gains for their clients in terms of independence, confidence and growth. Again this corresponds with the care (Table 10.5) that CPNs gave their clients. CPNs therefore had a mainly medical and psychological orientation to both their philosphical orientation and their practice. This approach also had more specific boundaries than was the case for CMs.

There were several areas of achievement that were mentioned by similar numbers of respondents from each of the three groups. These areas tended to be vaguer, such as 'quality of life in general'. Others of these areas tended to focus on the process of care delivery, such as building empathic relationships, as opposed to achieving client outcomes. Finally, several respondents talked of either having no expectations or of the need to have very modest expectations of process. Our earlier interviews (Repper, Ford and Cooke, 1994) found that CMs adopted an approach which set low expectations so that both client and CM could have greater chances of positive feedback.

From CMs' and CPNs' own reports there are obvious commonalities and overlaps between the two roles. However, CMs appear to have a more social role whereas CPNs relate a more medical and psychological orientation. These orientations are unbounded in the case of CMs while having professional demarcation for CPNs.

Client rights and creating dependency

A concern for case managers was that they might be restricting the client's right to refuse a service. In practice this issue had to be balanced against the case manager's responsibility to provide a service to clients who may be at risk of neglect, self injury or harming others. Case managers were able to remain sensitive to their clients' wishes; an important aim as they wished to build long-term supportive relationships.

All but four CMs and one CPN recognized that they could put too much time into their work with each individual client (Q3.6). While all groups felt that the consequence of putting in too much time would be client dependency on the worker the interpretation of the term dependency was quite different for the two groups. A CPN said: 'I have felt a little uncomfortable with the way they [CMs] work. I think to reinstitutionalize a group of people who are damaged because of being institutionalized isn't healthy and I think they [CMs] fall into the trap of doing so much so often that the person just reproduces his institutionalization and never moves on.' However, a CM had an alternative attitude towards doing a lot for clients: 'I bring her for her injection because she can never get up in time. A lot of people would contradict with that and say it's up to them to get themselves up. But that's not the way we look at it. We say it's important that she has the injection and that's the priority. How we get her there is not so important.' The same CM also argued that some degree of dependency was beneficial for people with a long-term mental illness so that service contact may be maintained.

The issues of client rights and dependency are both to do with balance. The balance between freedom and independence on the one hand with safety and avoiding negligence on the other. While both groups recognized this balance, the responses given by CMs suggest that their style of working and philosophical orientation, with its emphasis on taking responsibility and ensuring that care is provided, is more attuned to current policy.

DISCUSSION

The sub-study presented here does of course have its limitations. The sample sizes are small and were accrued from available staff rather than by random selection. Furthermore, there were few opportunities to control for workers having different case mixes of clients. The use of intensive semi-structured interviewing does however allow several important domains of the differences in ways of working between the groups to be unearthed.

CMs have not just expanded the role of the CPN. The orientation of the CM role is quite different, as it is explicitly based on client needs, whatever they may be. In this the CM role is anti-professional and unbounded. CMs also work with a broader spectrum of issues. Most noticeably they work in areas that would usually be described as social care. While working in these areas CMs do not negate health care needs, rather they see the provision of social care as a means towards the ends of providing health care.

The rationale behind the CM role is also different. The CM places less emphasis on client independence and more on making sure that appropriate care is provided. Also, the CM not only works as part of a team but sees her or himself as the centre of the team, often taking responsibility for arranging, monitoring and reviewing care.

Analysis of symptomatic and social functioning client outcomes from the RDP/DoH study provided a mixed group of results (Ford *et al.*, 1994b). The most likely explanation is that linking clients to medical services can increase appropriate take-up of medication services and hence improve acute symptoms. Equally, linking clients to rehabilitation services can improve social functioning and more persistent negative symptoms. The sub-study here has also shown how CMs placed considerable emphasis on improving the conditions that allow clients to make contact with appropriate services.

CONCLUSION

For nurses working in many new settings and in an increasing diversity of roles there are two conclusions that can be drawn from this sub-study. First, by virtue of extensive training in the mental health field and through considerable experience of working with people with the most distressing and disabling mental illnesses, nurses may be well equipped for the CM role. However, to develop into the CM role they will need to abandon the professional shackles that may impede the provision of client-centred care.

Secondly, the outcome results of the DoH/RDP Case Management Project suggest that case management may be necessary to make the link between clients and services. However, case management is not sufficient, in and of itself, to bring about improvements in mental state or social functioning. Specialist treatment and rehabilitative service are also needed. Therefore, there remains a clear role for nurses to deliver specific interventions that have demonstrable clinical or rehabilitative efficacy.

The ideal for clients with multiple and complex needs will be to receive the best of both worlds. The case manager acts as the 'travel guide' to negotiate, in full collaboration with the client, the often confusing network of professional and naturally occurring care. The professional nurse, through research and subsequent accredited training, is engaged to provide specific and effective interventions.

ACKNOWLEDGEMENTS

This work was funded by grants from the Research and Development for Psychiatry trustees and from the Department of Health. Research supervision for this paper was provided by Professor T. Craig, St Thomas', Professor J. Brooking, University of Birmingham and Mr P. Ryan, RDP.

REFERENCES

Barratt, E. (1989) community psychiatric nurses: their self-perceived roles. *Journal of Advanced Nursing*, **14**, 42–8.
Davidge, M., Elias, S., Jayes, B. *et al.* (1993) *Survey of English Mental Illness Hospitals*, Health Services Management Centre, Birmingham.
Department of Health (DoH) (1989). *Caring for People: Community Care in the Next Decade and Beyond*, HMSO, London.
Department of Health (DoH) (1990) *The Care Programme Approach for People with a Mental Illness Referred to the Specialist Psychiatric Services*, (HC(90)23), Department of Health, London.
Department of Health (DoH) (SSI). (1991) *Care Management and Assessment: Manager's Guide*, HMSO, London.
Department of Health (DoH) (1993) *Legislation Planned to Provide for Supervised Discharge of Psychiatric Patients*, (H93/908), Press Release, 12 August 1993.
Ford, R., Cooke, A. and Repper, J. (1992) Making a point of contact. *Nursing Times*, **88**, 40–2.
Ford, R., Repper, J., Cooke, A. *et al.* (1993a) *Implementing Case Management*, Research and Development for Psychiatry, London.

194   *Mental health nursing and case management*

Ford, R., Beadsmoore, A., Norton, P. *et al*. (1993b) Developing case management for the long-term mentally ill. *Psychiatric Bulletin*, **17**, 409–11.

Ford, R., Beadsmoore, A., Repper, J. *et al*. (1994a) Assertive outreach for people with a long-term mental illness: a multi-centre 30 month follow-up study, in submission.

Ford, R., Beadsmoore, A., Sutton, F. *et al*. (1994b) Outcomes of the case management project, in submission.

Pollock, L. (1988) The work of community psychiatric nursing. *Journal of Advanced Nursing*, **13**, 537–45.

Pollock, L. (1990) The goals and objectives of community psychiatric nursing, in *Community Psychiatric Nursing: a Research Perspective*, (ed. C. Brooker), Chapman & Hall, London.

Rapp, C. (1993) The strengths perspective of case management with persons suffering from severe mental illness, in *The Strengths Model of Social Work: Power in the People*, (ed. D. Saleebey), Longman, New York.

Repper, J., Ford, R. and Cooke, A. (1994) How can nurses build trusting relationships with people who have severe and long-term mental health problems? Experiences of case managers and their clients (accepted by *Journal of Advanced Nursing*).

Ryan, P., Ford, R. and Clifford, P. (1991) *Case Management and Community Care*, Research and Development for Psychiatry, London.

Stein, L.I. and Test, M.A. (1982) Community treatment of the young adult patient, in *New Directions for Mental Health Services 14*, (eds B. Pepper and Ryglewicz), Jossey-Bass, San Francisco.

Tyrer, P., Hawksworth, J., Hobbs, R. *et al*. (1990) The role of the community psychiatric nurse. *British Journal of Hospital Medicine*, **43**, 439–42.

White, E. (1990) Surveying CPNs. *Nursing Times*, **86**, 62–4.

Wooff, K., Goldberg, D.P. and Fryers, T. (1988) The practice of community psychiatric nursing and mental health social work in Salford: some implications for community care. *British Journal of Psychiatry*, **152**, 728–92.

CHAPTER ELEVEN

Intensive CPN community support for people with severe mental health problems in Greenwich

Margaret Cooney, Matt Muijen and
Geraldine Strathdee

INTRODUCTION

The White Paper *Caring for People* (HMSO, 1989) emphasized coordinated aftercare and care management as key elements in the care of patients with serious and long-term mental health problems. This was also addressed by the Care Programme Approach, which aimed to ensure that a multidisciplinary assessment was undertaken on all people with serious mental health problems discharged to or living in the community. In practice CPNs, being the link between hospital and community, are likely to be key workers in the majority of cases.

Generic CPNs are at risk of working in isolation, unable to offer well coordinated care to their often large caseloads (Wooff and Goldberg, 1988) which can also show a drift towards people with minor mental health problems. The lack of supervision and coordinated care might lead to poor services for patients with the greatest needs, specifically those with a severe and persistent mental illness. The importance of continuity of care and coordination of services (Bachrach, 1980, 1981) has been illustrated by studies reporting on the lack of planning at discharge, loss to follow-up, continuing presence of psychopathology, high readmission rates and poor psychosocial support provided by standard hospital-based services (Meltzer *et al.*, 1991; Wasylenki *et al.*, 1985). Multidisciplinary teams in which CPNs form the majority

of team members, or single disciplinary teams, have in a few cases concentrated on this group, aiming to improve their quality of life by offering
an alternative to standard outpatient care. Core elements of the approach
in these programmes were continuity of care and techniques of case
management.

The number of CPNs has increased considerably (White, 1990), but
favoured models of service delivery have not emerged yet in the UK. Generic
primary-care-based CPNs, CPNs as members of hospital teams,
multidisciplinary community teams combining crisis intervention and long-
term care, specialist CPN and specialist social worker teams can all be
responsible for the long-term mentally ill, either exclusively or as part of a
mixed caseload. How to use the CPN both effectively and efficiently is of
concern to providers and purchasers of community health services. Different
models of care need to be evaluated and set up in response to the type of
client the service is targeting.

In order to develop community service for the mentally ill, the client type
being targeted needs to be clarified. CPN's deal primarily with three broad
types of client: the elderly, people with psychological distress and long-term
clients. These three are not mutually exclusive but those with a persistent
and severe mental health problem are of major concern for several reasons.
Firstly, these people are often severely affected by their condition and are
dependent on intensive and continuing support for their survival in the
community. Secondly, they are heavy users of inpatient services, which is
very costly. CPN input may enable cheaper community living without reducing
quality of life. Thirdly, there is considerable social pressure for special attention
to this group, as often as not based on a dubious sense of danger.

In the past these long-term clients were at high risk of neglect, and were
only offered any input during a crisis, which often led to hospital admission.
Originally the role of the CPN was to 'support' discharged psychiatric
patients (May and Moore, 1963). The CPN made sure that patients were
taking their medication and sometimes discussed overall treatment plans with
a carer. In 1968 only 42 out of the then 2800 CPNs practised rehabilitation,
defined as teaching people to live in the community. Most remaining CPNs
were focusing on injections and day care.

Recently, specialist teams have been emerging, aiming to care for such
people. This chapter reports on the development of a CPN service in the
Greenwich Health Authority set up to meet the needs of people with severe
and persistent mental health problems in the community. The team was
evaluated and the intensive interventions of the community support team (CST)
were compared with standard generic input for the same client group.

The team was set up in response to policy changes aimed at the development of community psychiatric services, since it appeared that generic services
were unable to reduce the need for inpatient beds with these clients in
Greenwich.

THE DEVELOPMENT OF THE COMMUNITY SUPPORT TEAM (CST)

The CST is a single disciplinary team of CPNs developed in November 1988 as a part of the expanding community psychiatric nursing service in the Greenwich Health Authority. It offered assessment, treatment and long-erm continuous care. The team aimed to work specifically with clients because the generic services felt unable to care, due to the severity and persistence of their problems and the intensity of need for social care and rehabilitation.

The service commenced with the intention that four CPNs in the CST with a caseload ratio of 1:10 would provide more time-intensive input than the generic CPNs. Added to the existing aims and objectives of the CPN service the CST was to engage in:

1. comprehensive and intensive network of support for clients with long-term health problems based on individual functioning and needs;
2. the development of effective alternatives to reduce both the frequency of hospitalization and duration of stay;
3. secondary and tertiary prevention with models of care designed to maximize functioning, reduce negative behaviour and symptomatology and assist clients' optimum level of independence;
4. playing a key part in client advocacy of care, coordination and joint working with all agencies involved in care packages;
5. promoting social functioning within clients' own environment;
6. developing social skills training to enable clients to cope more effectively within their own daily living milieu.

To achieve this the team was located initially in an office where a weekly meeting was held on Monday morning to discuss diaries for the week. The policy of regular joint visits made team members aware of each other's clients, with the added benefit of safety. This policy later became more selective and was applied to acutely disturbed clients only. A business meeting was held weekly to discuss new ideas and developments within the service. The team provided a service 9 a.m. to 5 p.m. Monday to Friday. However, working times and practices were flexible according to needs. For example, because of a small caseload the service was able to respond quickly and spend time with a client in crisis.

Community psychiatric nursing services and referrals in Greenwich

In 1984, the community psychiatric nursing service consisted of two CPNs. In 1990 it had increased to 22, split across generic CPNs, the CST (four CPNs and four generic mental health workers), substance abuse (four) and the elderly (five CPNs and two mental health workers). Referrals to CPN services had increased from 315 in 1984 to 1361 in 1990, with the alcohol team receiving

253, the generic team 684, the EMI 324 and the CST 100. The generic service worked closely with GPs and were able to take self-referrals. Generic referrals came from consultants in 14%, the GP in 64% and elsewhere in 22%. Reasons for referrals were depression in 40%, 20% anxiety and 3% psychotic problems. This differs greatly from the CST, who received almost 100% psychotic clients with a long-term problem. CST referrals were accepted only from psychiatric services. This included consultants, generic CPNs, the ward staff, psychiatric social workers and the psychology department. All other agencies wishing to refer to the CST had to do so via specialist mental health services.

Intervention offered

Treatment and cure was seen to be an unrealistic objective. The approach was to focus on long-term maintenance and the development of positive coping mechanisms. Small, achievable goals were set specific to the individual client. The client group included the most dependent and disabled people living in the community most of whom had been in contact with services for long periods. However, they were often reluctant to engage with staff and viewed CPNs with suspicion. Commonly, the short-term goal was to get past the front door, from which point the emphasis was placed on what the individual wanted to be considered. Once a rapport and trust had been established the nurse would take on the role of client advocate and became involved in assessing needs and accessing the appropriate services.

Assessments were based on the aim for clients to function in their own environment. The effectiveness and appropriateness of interventions were assessed at 3-monthly intervals. If a client was deemed to require CST care but refused contact, the client was to be kept on the CPN caseload for 3 months, with monthly visits, after which time they would be put on the inactive list.

Once a client was accepted generally a comprehensive care package was offered. Many interventions were targeted towards daily living skills, including social skills training aimed at cooking, cleaning, shopping and budgeting. With the help of a fund raised by the CST some money was available for crisis periods, when benefits had not become available. Christmas was a period when funds were in great demand. The CST also developed a range of activities for clients. It set up a sports afternoon at the local leisure centre where people from the wards, as well as those in the community, played with staff on a informal basis (Bell and Cooney, 1993). This activity was felt to be beneficial to clients, with an average weekly attendance of 15. A drop-in centre was also established on a twice-weekly basis with the help of a generic CPN, but run by the service users.

Differences between interventions offered by the CST and generic teams

The CST and generic CPNs differed fundamentally in their working practices on at least three points. Firstly, the CST team offered a much more comprehensive and intensive service, allowed by the higher staff–patient ratio. Secondly, the type of client was different. The CST took referrals from the psychiatric service only while the generic CPNs worked closely with GPs, who were responsible for many of their referrals (64%). Generic CPNs had a mixed caseload from both primary care and specialist referral sources, with only 14.5% being under the care of a consultant psychiatrist. Thirdly, the CST did not discharge clients who were difficult to engage or were non-compliant with treatment, as was standard practice in the generic service. Put differently, the generic CPNs filtered out the most difficult clients while the CST specifically included them.

Tasks undertaken by the CST and the generic CPNs teams differed greatly (Table 11.1). Many patients in contact with the generic CPNs were administered medication, mainly depots. Although all CST patients received medication, many of those in CST care also received a wide range of additional interventions. As expected, the differences across the groups in amount of social interventions such as help with housing, financial and legal problems were large, but even the number of patients receiving medication favoured the CST. The generic nurses were providing counselling and medication as their main interventions with clients, with few of the social areas of need covered. The CST was offering 'problem solving', while relatively many clients in the generic group were given 'counselling', probably reflecting a difference in approach rather than in practice. The CST had included in their work remit to act with clients in a problem-solving manner, whereas the generic nurses were likely to provide 'problem solving' under the label of 'counselling'.

Table 11.1 Type of services CPNs engage in over the 18 months

	CST (n = 41)	Generic (n = 41)
Medication	41	28
Finance	28	5
Housing	33	5
Legal	18	0
Family support	40	8
Problem solving	50	11
Counselling	23	24

Although the CST and CPNs were involved in all aspects of care the role of medication was felt to be important and a means of ensuring that a person could live in the community. It was found that of those clients who required hospital care 72% had refused their medication within 3 months of being readmitted. Much of the CST's time was spent on trying to convince clients to take medication to prevent them becoming unwell.

The CST included techniques that are now a common part of the Care Programme Approach, including social and medical issues. A part of the case management approach was that clients would have a named worker who would be the coordinator of social and health care. Although the CST were acting in the spirit of case management there were fundamental differences. They had no training in case management techniques such as need assessments or interagency liaison and were forced to act for clients themselves due to a lack of other services in the borough. Other studies on the effectiveness of case management report that positive outcomes are likely to be dependent on the additional local resources (Chapter 10). Although assumed to act as case managers, the CST team functioned more like client advocates.

Number of contacts with clients

Number of contacts of each of the teams shows some interesting differences (Table 11.2). Numbers of staff in the teams were comparable but, considering the small caseload of the CST staff, the CST were obviously putting in many more visits than the generic team. On average the CST had four times as many client contacts as the generic team.

Table 11.2 Number of clients' contacts with the CST and generic CPN teams

	No. of direct contacts
Generic	3227
EMI	3925
CST	3132
Drug	566
Alcohol	1433
Total	12 283

A major difference between the two groups was continuity of care over the 18 month period (Figure 11.1). This shows that most contacts occurred during the initial 6 months in the CST group, while number of contacts remained constant in the generic care group. At no point was the number of generic

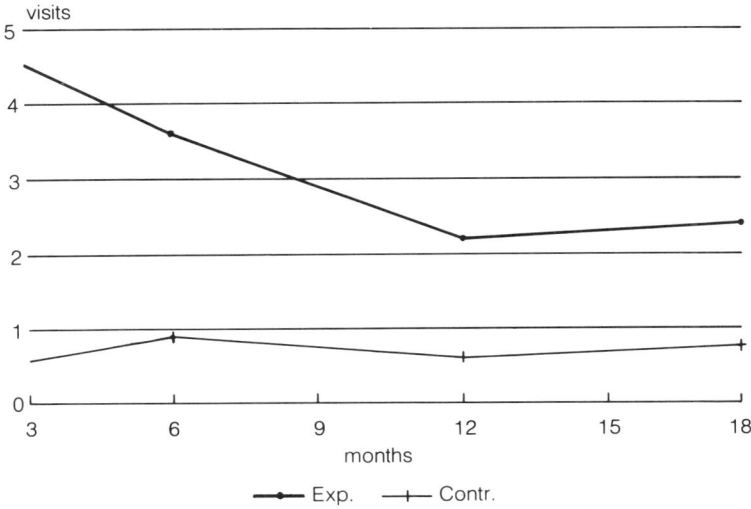

Figure 11.1 Number of visits in the experimental and control groups.

contacts even 50% of the number in the CST group, indicating the far greater continuity as well as intensity of the CST group.

Receiving a referral in the generic services does not always result in a subsequent visit. If an outpatients appointment is made and not attended, a generic nurse may discharge that person from his/her caseload. In contrast, the CST nurses did thorough assessments of all referrals and did not discharge people. The high number of contacts in the CST was only made possible because of small caseloads, a key principle of case management. It is generally recognized that case management cannot work well when the number of clients is more than 15, because of the intensity of the work.

OUTCOMES FOR CLIENTS AS PART OF THE EVALUATION STUDY

Effectiveness of the CST and the generic teams were evaluated in considerable detail. The hypothesis was that:

1. a CPN team using a comprehensive aftercare service improves status, social functioning, patient satisfaction and family burden of chronic psychotic patients as compared to generic CPN care;
2. such a service reduces the number and duration of admissions to hospital.

Clients were randomized to either the CST or the generic team on discharge from Greenwich District Hospital. Each group included 41 clients. To ensure that only clients with long-term health needs in the community were included, entry criteria to the study were:

1. a diagnosis of a psychotic disorder (schizophrenia or affective disorder);
2. a duration of illness of more than 2 years;
3. at least two admissions in the past 2 years;
4. residence in the Greenwich Health Authority area.

Each person was assessed at four times: at baseline or entry into the study and at 6, 12 and 18 months. Data were obtained on clinical status, social functioning and user and family satisfaction. At entry into the study, service use data were collected retrospectively for the past 3 months. At subsequent interviews, service use was obtained for the period between interviews. Data were also collected on frequency and duration of CPN input including office hours and domiciliary visits.

Characteristics of these clients are shown in Table 11.3. It can be seen that the two groups of clients were relatively similar, the majority being diagnosed with schizophrenia although slightly more of the generic clients were diagnosed as suffering with mania. There was a slightly higher proportion

Table 11.3 Client characteristics (from Muijen *et al.*, 1994)

Characteristic	CST (n = 41)	Generic (n = 41)
Mean age (SD)	38(12)	36(10)
Male (% in parentheses)	25(56)	23(56)
Diagnosis (% in parentheses)		
Schizophrenia	35(85)	33(80)
Mania	3(7)	7(17)
Psychotic depression	3(7)	1(3)
Mean no. days in hospital before study	232	232
Mean no. admissions before study	5.4	6.0
Living situation (% in parentheses)		
Alone	25(61)	16(36)
With spouse/child	14(33)	15(37)
Sheltered accommodation	1(2)	9(22)
Not known	1(2)	1(2)
Ethnicity (% in parentheses)		
UK/Irish	27(66)	31(66)
African/Afro-Caribbean	12(29)	7(17)
Asian	1(2)	2(5)
Other	1(2)	1(2)

of clients living on their own in the CST. Although these differences in baseline characteristics were not significant, some bias cannot be excluded, due to the relatively small numbers. Significantly more clients in the generic group lived in sheltered or staffed accommodation ($p = 0.01$) and, since living with support can be a good predictor of outcome, this could lead to favourable results for the generic team. Therefore, this was taken into account in the analysis by stratifying for this variable.

Clinical outcomes

The main objective of this study was to explore whether the CST, by using an individualized and need-led form of care and offering a comprehensive range of care, would improve clinical status and functioning and consequently reduce the number and duration of admissions to hospitals.

Table 11.4 shows that none of the ratings scales suggests significant changes in either group. The PSE (Wing, Cooper and Sartorius, 1974), and BPRS (Overall and Gorham, 1962) both measure psychopathology, and after 18 months neither group had improved in this area. This should not come

Table 11.4 Means and standard errors of rating scales

	Baseline		*18 months*	
	Experimental (s.e.) n	*Control (s.e.) n*	*Experimental (s.e.) n*	*Control (s.e.) n*
GAS	45.8 (2.0) 40	40.9 (2.2) 38	42.6 (2.4) 31	39.3 (2.8) 27
PSE (total)	15.4 (2.5) 39	20.1 (3.1) 37	20.3 (2.6) 28	27.6 (4.7) 25
BPRS	43.4 (2.1) 40	43.6 (2.3) 38	44.4 (2.4) 31	51.8 (3.7) 26
SAS	3.7 (0.2) 37	3.9 (0.3) 33	3.6 (0.3) 24	4.2 (0.3) 22
Patient satisfaction	n/a		26.4 (1.5) 23	23.9 (2.0) 14
Relative satisfaction	n/a		54.9 (2.4) 15	55.3 (1.9) 10

as a surprise, since people had entered the study on discharge from hospital, i.e. when in a relatively good condition. Social functioning, as measured by the Social Adjustment Scale (SAS) (Weissman *et al.*, 1971), had also changed little. The Global Assessment Scale (GAS) can be regarded as a summary scale, scoring in a single number symptomatology and functioning, and its scores are consistent with the other scales (on the GAS and the satisfaction scales higher scores indicate improvement, on the other scales deterioration).

Some subgroups were considered separately. It will be remembered that generic clients lived in residential care. No difference in outcome in any area was found for this group, however, either at baseline or at follow-up.

Social functioning

The lack of improvement in social functioning is particularly disappointing. The score on the SAS indicates that these clients were moderately impaired (maximum score $= 7$) and there was very little, if any, improvement in social functioning over the 18-month period. The SAS covers the areas of work, social outlets, the extended family, partnerships, relationships with parents and the family unit and economic status.

Very few in the sample were in any paid employment, which is unfortunately typical of this client group. Almost all clients depended for the bulk of their income on DSS benefits, with the occasional person receiving additional monies from relatives or spouses. Over the 18 months four out of 41 (10%) of clients in the CST were in any employment of any stage. One was a full-time welder, one a part-time kitchen assistant, another an administrative assistant and the final person did labouring work. Only one client described herself as being a housewife. Although many were at home much of the time they were more likely to label themselves as being registered unemployed, or even not working and yet not registered as unemployed. Only 13% were registered as unemployed and 71% were unregistered. This indicates that many people with mental health problems are not working and not registered, a large body of hidden unemployment.

In the generic group a slightly higher proportion were in some form of employment (seven out of 41, 17%). Two were in sheltered employment; one each worked as a road sweeper, a lift maintenance engineer, a full-time market researcher, in a central London shop and in a restaurant. Only 5% of this group were registered as unemployed and 70% were not registered whilst not working.

Whether they are registered as unemployed or not, the vast majority of clients were not working and thus heavily reliant on social security benefit payments. Only one CST person was not in receipt of DSS benefits as her husband was her source of income; none in the generic team received money from partners. The average level of benefit received, excluding housing benefit was £43.60.

Clients' and relatives' satisfaction

Only those clients and their relatives in contact with the services during the preceding 6 months were rated at each period, using the Client Satisfaction Scale (Larsen *et al.*, 1979). Client satisfaction remained very stable throughout the study. Clients in both groups who received services were satisfied with the quality of care they received.

Relatives' satisfaction was very similar across the groups at each point. Satisfaction increased somewhat between 6 and 12 months into the study, especially in the generic group. Numbers in this group were very low, however. It appears that those who had contact with CPNs were as satisfied as those who had no contact.

These results are disappointing as well as surprising, although not dissimilar from other work (Muijen *et al.*, 1992, a, b). Can we really accept that clients and carers are equally satisfied with a need-led and comprehensive care approach as with a minimal input or little input at all? This clearly questions either the validity of the ratings or the working methods of the CST. This will be further explored later on.

Hospital, psychiatrist and GP use

The intensive work of the CST was expected to reduce hospital use, preferably both numbers of admissions and length of stay. The impact on hopsital use was disappointing, however. During the 18-month period, the 41 CST clients had been admitted an average of 0.4 times (s.e. 0.1) for a mean duration of 14.9 days (s.e. 5 days) as compared to respectively 0.3 admissions (0.1) and 15.6 days (6.2) for the generic clients. Clearly, neither the number of admissions nor the duration of stay was significantly different between the CST and the generic clients support team.

The involvement of psychiatrists and GPs was remarkably similar across the groups, although variations among individual patients was considerable. CST patients were seen by psychiatrists on average seven times and generic clients six times over 18 months. GPs saw CST clients 2.5 times and generic clients four times during this time. To put it differently, psychiatrists saw these patients, with very severe problems, on average every 2.5–3 months and GPs had even less frequent contact.

COST

The cost effectiveness of a service is increasingly important since service providers and purchasers have limited resources which have to be spent on the most effective and efficient resources. The interpretation of this study will have to balance clinical effectiveness with user and carer satisfaction and cost. Costs are a somewhat flexible concept, and boundaries have to be determined. We will distinguish direct costs to the health services, social services and housing. This analysis was undertaken by the PSSRU (McCrone, Beecham and Knapp, 1994).

The health services costs were higher for CST patients, as can be expected since these clients received considerably more input from CPNs and an equal number of bed-days. Health service costs were about £195 weekly for CST clients and £155 for generic clients. The large majority of these costs were hospital costs, with only £12 versus £3 respectively spent weekly on CPN care. Social service costs were about equal, at £12 weekly. The main cost difference was due to the greater use of hostels in the generic group. This meant that weekly accommodation costs were £120 for CST clients and £220 for generic clients. Consequently, total costs favoured the CST. Over 18 months the CST clients cost on average £89 a week less than the generic clients.

Accommodation accounted for 52% of the total costs for the CST client and 70% of the generic client costs. Accommodation costs invariably constitute the greatest element in a cost package. As more people were in staffed accommodation in the generic team this elevated their total costs. It should be remembered, however, that considerably more generic clients lived in residential care on entry and this has not been considered in the cost analysis. This makes a firm conclusion haphazard. Health service costs were higher in the CST, while total costs were lower, largely due to a factor that was somewhat confounded. It should not be ignored, however, that more people in the generic group required residential care in the process of this study. This suggests that a proportion of the accommodation saving in the CST group was the result of the intensive support. What proportion is unclear.

ISSUES ARISING FROM THE CST PERSPECTIVE

The working practices of the CST created consistency and continuity within aftercare, often eliminating the traditional barriers across the sectors which jointly provide mental health. The nurse became a friendly, dependable advocate sticking with the person through good and difficult times, when many of the other health and social professions would not have been available.

The results showed no difference in the recorded number of hospital admissions between the two groups. Sometimes such figures hide important variations, though. For example, they did not indicate that 72% of the CST admissions were nurse-aided, while only 20% of the generic admissions were instigated by a CPN. This emphasizes the key importance of monitoring people in the community and the importance that was placed on keeping the individual safe. A hospital admission was not necessarily seen as a failure but as potential support for the client who became aware of such health needs at the time.

CST clients over time became less resistant to being admitted and would occasionally ask to be sent to the ward instead of requiring a compulsory mental health section.

The fact that the CST had close links with the ward staff meant that admissions were often smooth and done quickly but once admitted the CPN had little say over treatment and discharge. The role of medication compliance needs to be stressed again as there is some relationship between those who were admitted and those who ceased their medication.

Although the CST nurses were no more successful than the generic CPNs in reducing hospital use, they did increase independent living. More of their clients stayed in their own homes with only two going into residential settings, whereas the generic group had 12 people over the 18 months living in hostels and three in the regional secure unit.

Keeping people in their own home was seen to be a success by the CST, improving social care and daily living skills and possibly increasing their standard of living and quality of life. Unfortunately, this was not measured, and it is unclear whether such improvements were achieved.

From working with this client group it is evident that loneliness and isolation were important factors affecting mental health; 61% of the CST clients were living alone whereas only 39% of the generic clients were living without others in their home. Time spent alone was a common feature, especially where individuals did not attend day centres or regular activities.

Despite the government directive of the Care Programme Approach, many individuals with long-term problems may refuse contacts. This highlights the need for (1) identifying those who will be difficult to engage with and (2) providing optimal services for those who do and do not agree to be involved with an intensive community service.

The results of this evaluation appear to be disappointing for intensive interventions applied to a client group with severe and persistent mental health problems. The findings raise a great deal of potential debate and controversy regarding what service planning or recommendations can be provided for such a vulnerable and difficult-to-engage group.

The following points have to be considered carefully before conclusions about this work lead to positive or negative action.

1. During the 18 months of evaluation a service in development was being evaluated, rather than a service working to its full potential. Staff had not been fully trained, if trained at all. It is unlikely that the results of this study represent the full potential effectiveness of community teams; they more closely reflect the minimum impact they can make.
2. Symptomatology of this client group cannot be expected to alter greatly and there will always be a need for inpatient beds. A preoccupation with bed usage may be unhelpful: at least as important are changes in standard of living and quality of a person's life.

3. Other services need to be available if a case management service is to function well. Moreover, multidisciplinary teams would be advantageous, rather than one discipline attempting to provide all the social and health interventions.
4. The CST provided 70% of all social care interventions with no input from social services. Joint working practices need to be developed between health and social services.
5. Community services should be more flexible with regard to working out of office hours. A range of intervention and activities are required, not only to deal with crises but also with the isolation and loneliness often felt by these clients in the evenings and at weekends.
6. The CPN is the link between the hospital and the community. It needs to be recognized that the CPN needs to be involved in the pre-discharge arrangements and the development of care programmes.
7. The criteria for intensive input needs to be clarified. Assessment of need and availability of individually suited care should be central to all care provision. Certain clients did well and others did not with the present services. The nurses, from a professional, subjective viewpoint, felt that the main issue was compliance or willingness to engage with services. It was noted that intensive interventions were only needed for 3–6 month periods. Once engagement had been established, maintenance contacts, e.g. visits on a monthly basis, sufficed.

DISCUSSION

This study compared a nursing team using a case management model with generic CPNs and found few results in favour of the case management team. Results of other studies were generally more positive with many finding reduced hospital use (Stein and Test, 1980; Hoult and Reynolds, 1983; Bond, Miller and Krumwied, 1988; Borland, McRae and Lycan, 1989; Wright *et al.*, 1989; Muijen *et al.*, 1992a, b), but not all (Goering *et al.*, 1988).

Several important differences exist between those evaluations and the present one. Patients generally suffered from more acute disorders than entered the present study, and were randomized at points in time when sympomatology and functioning were at their worst, allowing major improvement, rather than at discharge as in this study when many patients were functioning at relatively high levels. Moreover, in contrast to the nurses in the present project, all other studies evaluated multidisciplinary teams including psychiatrists, social workers and occupational therapists.

Several important questions remain unanswered by any studies investigating community support. The intensity and duration of care required for the best result is unknown (Borland, McRae and Lycan, 1989). Future research needs to focus on this balance, since it is not realistic to expect specialist teams to care for small groups of patients for decades on end. Another important question is which clients are most likely to improve most with intensive aftercare. Some clients did benefit both in their health and in their overall wellbeing from the CST input but because of the diverse sociodemographic backgrounds of people included and the large variation of outcomes in both treatment groups such subgroups were impossible to identify.

An explanation for the similar outcome despite different amounts of input may be that the generic clients were receiving support from others such as social and voluntary services. Both groups in this study had equal access to day care and some other forms of support, although the availability of such support was limited. Community care depends on a minimum number of resources and the efficient functioning of community facilities. If no support services are available, coordination of care is difficult and the key worker needs to concentrate on direct interventions. This is likely to produce demoralization as well as role confusion and burn-out in unsupported teams. CPNs had some problems obtaining the appropriate back-up services and this may have impaired effectiveness depsite them remaining keen and motivated in their dealings with clients.

The number of psychiatrists and psychologists was well below recommended national norms and staff with rehabilitation skills were unavailable in the district. This absence of multidisciplinary team work and skills may have also reduced effectiveness.

Finally, training is essential. Unless the skills of case management will be taught, it cannot be expected to be effective. And unless the willingness is there to make such investment, it cannot be hoped that community care will benefit those suffering from the most severe mental health problems.

REFERENCES

Bachrach, L.L. (1980) Overview: model programs for chronic mental patients. *American Journal of Psychiatry*, **137**, 1023–31.

Bachrach, L.L. (1981) Continuity of care for chronic mental patients: a conceptual analysis. *American Journal of Psychiatry*, **138**, 1449–55.

Bell, R. and Cooney, M. (1993) Sorting chances. *Nursing Times*, **89**, 62–3.

Bond, G.R., Miller, R.D. and Krumwied, R.D. (1988) Assertive case management in three CMHCs: a controlled study. *Hospital and Community Psychiatry*, **39**, 411–18.

Borland, A., McRae, J. and Lycan, C. (1989) Outcomes of five years of continuous intensive case management. *Hospital and Community Psychiatry*, **40**, 369–76.

Goering, P.N., Wasylenki, D.A., Farkas, M. *et al.* (1988) What difference does case management make? *Hospital and Community Psychiatry*, **39**, 272–6.

HMSO (1989) *Caring for People: Community Care in the Next Decade and Beyond*, Cmnd 849, HMSO, London.

Hoult, J. and Reynolds, I. (1983) *Psychiatric Hospital versus Community Treatment: a controlled study*, Department of Health, New South Wales.

Larsen, D.H., Atkinson, C.C., Hargreaves, W.A. and Nguyen, T.D. (1979) Assessment of client/patient satisfaction: development of a general scale. *Evaluation and Program Planning*, **2**, 197–207.

May, A. and Moore, S. (1963) The mental health nurse in the community. *Lancet*, **i**, 213–14.

McCrone, P., Beecham, J. and Knapp, M. (1994) Community psychiatric nurses in an intensive community support team: comparisons with generic CPN care. *British Journal of Psychiatry*, **165**, 218–21.

Meltzer, D., Hale, A.S., Malik, S.H. *et al.* (1991) Community care for patients with schizophrenia one year after hospital discharge. *British Medical Journal*, **303**, 1023–6.

Muijen, M., Marks, I.M., Connolly, J. *et al.* (1992a) The Daily Living Program: Preliminary comparison of community versus hospital based treatment for the seriously mentally ill facing emergency admission. *British Journal of Psychiatry*, **160**, 379–83.

Muijen, M., Marks, I., Connolly, J. and Audini, B. (1992b) Home based care and standard hospital care for patients with severe mental illness: a randomised controlled trial. *British Medical Journal*, **304**, 749–54.

Muijen, M., Cooney, M., Strathdee, G. *et al.* (1994) A randomized controlled study of an intensive support CPN team versus generic CPN care for long-term mentally ill patients in the Greenwich district. *British Journal of Psychiatry* (in press).

Overall, J.E. and Gorham, D.R. (1962) The Brief Psychiatric Rating Scale. *Psychological Reports*, **10**, 799–812.

Stein, L.J. and Test, M.A. (1980) Alternative to mental hospital treatment. 1, Conceptual model, treatment program and clinical evaluation. *Archives of General Psychiatry*, **37**, 392–7.

Wasylenki, D., Goering, P., Lancee, W. *et al.* (1985) Psychiatric aftercare in a metropolitan setting. *Canadian Journal of Psychiatry*, **30**, 329–36.

Weissman, M.M., Paykel, E.S., Siegel, R. and Klerman, G. (1971) The social role performance of depressed women: comparisons with a normal group. *American Journal of Orthopsychiatry*, **41**, 390–405.

White, E. (1990) Surveying CPNs. *Nursing Times*, **86**, 62–6.

Wing, J.K., Cooper, J.E. and Sartorius, N. (1974) *The Description and Classification of Psychiatric Symptoms: an Instruction Manual for the PSE and Catego System*. Cambridge University Press, Cambridge.

Wooff, K. and Goldberg, D.P. (1988) Further observations on the practice of community care in Salford. *British Journal of Psychiatry*, **153**, 30–7.

Wright, R.G., Heiman, J.R., Shupe, J. and Olvera, G. (1989) Defining and measuring stabilization of patients during 4 years of intensive community support. *American Journal of Psychiatry*, **146**, 1293–8.

CHAPTER TWELVE

Community psychiatric nursing: a selected bibliography
Edward White

INTRODUCTION

The belief that a free-standing community psychiatric nursing biblio-graphy would be a welcome inclusion to a text book dedicated to the same subject took root in 1990. At that time, the present writer was the Research Advisor to the Community Psychiatric Nurses Association (CPNA). Mindful of the volume and nature of the enquiries he dealt with in that capacity, he published a research-note in the journal of the CPNA (White, 1990) to draw attention to two preliminary steps which novice community psychiatric nurse (CPN) researchers should take before his advice was sought.

Firstly, he advised prospective enquirers to write to him, rather than telephone. This, he argued, was because often 'something had not been thought about, until it had been written upon'. Most enquirers had not done so before contact was made. Secondly, because most enquirers were innocent, he recommended them to read, at the very least, Brooker, C. (ed.) (1990) *Community Psychiatric Nursing: a Research Perspective*, vol. 1, Chapman & Hall, London; Marsh, C. (1982) *The Survey Method: the Contribution of Surveys to Sociological Explanation*, George Allen & Unwin, London; and Lofland, J. and Lofland, L. (1984) *Analysing Social Settings*, 2nd edn, Wadworth. Other texts might now be added, 5 years on, not least Brooker, C. and White, E. (eds) (1990) *Community Psychiatric Nursing: a Research Perspective*, vol 2, Chapman & Hall, London, though Marsh, 1982 and Lofland and Lofland, 1984, would still be important as introductory readers. This suggestion was to give naive enquirers a feel for, though clearly not a command of, some of the issues involved in empirical work. It was not unusual to learn that

212 *Community psychiatric nursing: selected bibliography*

they had severely limited time, no money and no access to other necessary resources. Sometimes, given these limitations, the intended projects were unrealistically ambitious; for example, a UK-wide postal survey was proposed as a basis for a 3000-word college essay.

White (1990) argued that many of the methodological and substantive enquiries he received from prospective CPN researchers would have been satisfactorily answered by an examination of an appropriate literature and, therefore, much of the proposed empirical work would be rendered unnecessary. This, he argued, would have a positive effect and should be welcomed because the task of locating and using the sound research findings was as crucial an activity as seeking to generate them.

The following bibliography contains 500 citations, the earliest of which is 1959. It has been guillotined at 1992. In the December of that year, Volume 2 of this series was published, although it appeared with a date of 1993. All references listed here, including those from Volume 2, were purposively selected for inclusion from a much larger bank held by the present writer, managed with the use of the American PAPYRUS Bibliography System (Research Software Design 1992). Thus, constrained by available space, this bibliography is not claimed to be exhaustive; indeed, it represents something less than half the references published on community psychiatric nursing over the same period.

The external data bases interrogated for this compilation included DHSS-Data; Health Care Database of the English National Board for Nursing, Midwifery and Health Visiting; Datastar; Dialog; Medline; CINAHL, together with an incorporation of the Biographical Series J5 of the Royal College of Nursing. The citations listed here have been organized into the broad subject categories of 'practice, 'education', 'organization' and 'other'. A sub-category of 'practice' has been created and labelled 'role'. In turn, 'role' has itself been sub-categorized into 'social worker' and 'general practitioner'. However, all such categories are not necessarily mutually exclusive because many of the publications, if not most, deal with issues which are not discrete to (say) practice or education. Within categories, citations have been arranged alphabetically by first author.

This bibliography is intended to assist both the prospective researcher and the interested reader to locate published material germane to community psychiatric nursing. In so doing, it is to be hoped that, by consulting the literature in a rational manner, readers might have their substantive questions answered. If they are not, new research proposals should be considered for development in the confident knowledge that rigorously supervised empirical work might then be justified. When such work has been conducted and written-up, it too should enter the public domain, whereupon it would become available for consideration of future revisions to this and other bibliographies.

REFERENCES

Research Software Design (1992) PAPYRUS Bibliography System, 2718 SW Kelly Street, Suite 181, Portland, OR 97201, USA.
White, E. (1990) Research. *Community Psychiatric Nursing Journal*, **10**, 38–9.

PRACTICE

Adams, T. (1987) How does it feel to be a caregiver? *Community Psychiatric Nursing Journal*, **7**(3), 11–17.
Adams, T. (1989) Growth of a speciality: strategies for CPNs working with elderly people. *Nursing Times*, **85**(40), 30–2.
Adams, T. (1990) Psychiatric nurse and community mental health. *Nursing Standard* **4**(37), 30–1.
Aiken, L. (1987) Unmet needs of the chronically mentally ill: will nursing respond? *Image: Journal of Nursing Scholarship*, **19**(3), 121–5.
Allan, A. (1988) No-show at a community mental health clinic: a pilot study. *International Journal of Social Psychiatry*, **34**(1), 40–6.
Allinson, M. (1984) Is the practice of community psychiatric nursing becoming too technical? *Community Psychiatric Nursing Journal*, **4**(6), 16–18.
Altschul, A. (1973) A multi-disciplinary approach to psychiatric nursing. *Nursing Times*, **69**(15), 508–11.
American Nurses Association (1970) Community mental health nursing. *American Journal of Nursing*, **May**, 1019–21.
Anonymous (1977) Community psychiatric nurses identify their own special skills. *Nursing Times*, **73**(22), 804.
Anonymous (1990) Standards for community pscyhiatric nursing services. *Community Psychiatric Nursing Journal*, **10**(4), 8–13.
Armitage, P. (1984) The community psychiatric nurse in California. *Nursing Times*, **80**(15), 38–9.
Armstrong, J. (1987) Community mental health nurses; frontline workers. *Canadian Journal of Psychiatric Nursing*, **28**(4), 4–6.
Atha, C. (1990) The role of the CPN with clients who deliberately harm themselves, in *Community Psychiatric Nursing: a Research Perspective*, (ed. C. Brooker), Chapman & Hall, London.
Baier, M. (1987) Case management with the chronically mentally ill. *Journal of Psychosocial Nursing and Mental Health Services*, **26**(7), 17–21.
Balestrieri, M. (1987) Long-stay and long-term psychiatric patients in an area with a community-based system of care: a register follow-up study (In Italy). *International Journal of Social Psychiatry*, **33**(4), 251–62.
Barker, A. and Black, S. (1971) An experiment in integrated psychogeriatric care. *Nursing Times*, **67**(45), 1395–9.
Battaglia, G. (1987) The expanding role of the nurse and the contracting role of the hospital in Italy. *International Journal of Social Psychiatry*, **33**(2), 115–18.
Bennett, C. (1989) The Worcester Development Project: general practitioner satisfaction with a new community psychiatric service. *Journal of the Royal College of General Practitioners*, **39**, 106–9.

Bennett, D. (1977) Kept in the community. *New Scientist*, **9 July**.

Black, S. and Simon, R. (1980) The specialist nurse, support care and the elderly mentally infirm. *Community Outlook*, **February**, 45–6.

Briscoe, M. and Wilkinson, G. (1989) General practitioners use of community psychiatric nursing services: a preliminary survey. *Journal of the Royal College of General Practitioners*, **49**, 412–14.

Brooke, A. and Haque, G. (1972) An aspect of community psychiatry. *General Practitioner Forum*, **209**, 89–94.

Brooker, C. (1985) Community mental health services in Italy: the implications for community psychiatric nurses in the United Kingdom. *Community Psychiatric Nursing Journal* **5**(3), 11–18.

Brooker, C. (1985) Two psychiatric entities: the community psychiatric nurse and the nurse therapist. *Nursing Mirror*, **160**(2), 35–6.

Brooker, C. (1986) Community psychiatric care: pragmatics and ethics. *British Journal of Hospital Medicine*, **36**(5), 321.

Brooker, C. (1988) Community psychiatric nursing and high expressed emotion. *Community Psychiatry: its Practice and Management*, **1**(1), 11–13.

Brooker, C. (ed.) (1990) *Community Psychiatric Nursing: a Research Perspective*, Chapman & Hall, London.

Brooker, C. (1990) Expressed emotion and psychosocial intervention: a review. *International Journal of Nursing Studies*, **27**(3), 267–76.

Brooker, C. (1990) Helping families cope with illness: the theory of expressed emotion. *Nursing Times*, **86**(2), 26–9.

Brooker, C. (1990) The skill of giving information and CPNs. *Nursing Standard*, **4**(22), 31–3.

Brooker, C. (1992) Community psychiatric nursing, in *A Textbook of Psychiatric Nursing*, (eds B. Thomas and S. Ritter), Churchill Livingstone, Edinburgh.

Brooker, C. and Baguley, I. (1990) Schizophrenia and sexual functioning. *Nursing Standard*, **4**(39), 34–5.

Brooker, C. and Baguley, I. (1990) SNAP decisions. *Nursing Times*, **86**(41), 56–8.

Brooker, C., Barrowclough, C. and Tarrier, N. (1992) Evaluating information given to CPNs to families caring for a relative with schizophrenia. *Journal of Clinical Nursing*, **1**(1), 19–25.

Brooker, C. and Jane, D. (1984) Time to re-think a community psychiatric nursing team. *Community Outlook*, **April**, 132–4.

Brooker, C. and White, E. (eds) (1993) *Community Psychiatric Nursing: A Research Perspective*, vol. 2, Chapman & Hall, London.

Brook, P. and Cooper, B. (1975) Community mental health care: primary team and specialist services. *Journal of the Royal College of General Practitioners*, **25**, 93–110.

Buller, S. (1989) Lasting attachments: how psychiatric nurse specialists can reduce the time GPs spend with mentally ill clients and the number of hospital admissions. *Nursing Times*, **85**(25), 36–7.

Burgoyne, G. (1990) The CPN and eating disorders. *Journal of Clinical Practice, Education and Management*, **4**(2), 30–2.

Burnard, P. (1988) Equality and meaning: issues in the interpersonal relationship. *Community Psychiatric Nursing Journal*, **8**(6), 17–21.

Burnard, P. and Morrison, P. (1989) CPNs attitudes to counselling. *Nursing Times*, **85**, 56.

Burns, T., Paykel, E., Ezekiel, A. and Lemon, S. (1988) Care of chronic neurotic out-patients by community psychiatric nurses: a long term follow-up study. *British Journal of Psychiatry*, **May**, 685–90.

Butterworth, C. (1979) Assessment and evaluation of patients by community psychiatric nurses. University of Aston, MSc Thesis.

Butterworth, C. (1989) Working for patients in a changing world. *Community Psychiatric Nursing Journal*, **9**(3), 22–3.

Butterworth, C. (1991) European nursing: meeting the challenge. *Community Psychiatric Nursing Journal*, **11**(3), 8–14.

Caldwell, J. (1989) *Community Psychiatric Nursing Survey on Behalf of the RCN CPN Forum*, Research Monograph, Royal College of Nursing, London.

Caldwell, J., Corrigan, J., Fagbadigun, R. *et al.* (1985) Good practices. *Community Psychiatric Nursing Journal*, **5**(1), 23–4.

Carlisle, D. (1990) Lockerbie one year on: three community psychiatric nurses involved with victims and rescuers. *Nursing Times*, **86**, 54–6.

Carson, J., Bartlett, H. and Croucher, P. (1991) Stress in community psychiatric nursing: a preliminary investigation. *Community Psychiatric Nursing Journal*, **11**(2), 8–12.

Chaloner, C. and Kinsella, C. (1992) Care with conviction: forensic community psychiatric nurses caring for mentally disordered offenders. *Nursing Times*, **22 April**, 50–2.

Channock, A. (1977) Essential skills of the CPN. *Nursing Mirror*, **145**(8), 12.

Clarke, J. (1976) Community psychiatric nursing. *JBCNS Supplement, Nursing Mirror*, **143**(6).

Clarke, M. (1980) Psychiatric liaison with health visitors. *Health Trends*, **12**, 98–100.

Clarke, M., Williams, A. and Jones, P. (1981) A psychogeriatric survey of old people's homes. *British Medical Journal*, **November**, 1307–10.

Collins-Colon, T. (1990) Do it yourself: medication management for community based clients. *Journal of Psychosocial Nursing and Mental Health Services*, **28**(6), 25–9.

Community Psychiatric Nurses Association (1978) *Responsibilities and Liabilities of Transporting Patients in the Community*, Community Psychiatric Nurses Association, Bristol.

Community Psychiatric Nurses Association (1983) *The Clinical Responsibilities of the CPN: A Discussion Document*, Community Psychiatric Nurses Association, Bristol.

Community Psychiatric Nurses Association (1985) *The Clinical Nursing Responsibilities of the Community Psychiatric Nurse*, CPNA Publications, Bristol.

Community Psychiatric Nurses Association (1988) *CPNA Directory of Innovative Practice*, CPNA Publications, Bradford.

Community Psychiatric Nurses Association (1989) *Moving Out: a Discussion on Resettlement Issues*, CPNA Publications, Bradford.

Community Psychiatric Nurses Association (1989) *Clinical Practice Issues*, vol. 1, CPNA Publications, Bradford.

Conhye, A. (1987) Hidden assets: study of GPs perceptions of community psychiatric nurses. *Nursing Times*, **83**, 49–50.

Cooling, A. (1978) Community psychiatric nursing, in *Contemporary Themes in Psychiatric Nursing*, (ed. H. Leopoldt), Squibb & Son, Twickenham.

Corea, S. (1987) Care of the elderly: joint CPNA/PNA discussion paper. *Community Psychiatric Nursing Journal*, **7**(2), 34–36.

Corrigan, J. and Soni, S. (1977) Community psychiatric nursing: an appraisal of its impact on community psychiatry in Manchester, England. *Journal of Advanced Nursing*, **2**, 347–54.

Crosby, R. (1987) Community care of the chronically mentally ill. *Journal of Psychosocial Nursing and Mental Health Services*, **25**(1), 33–7.

Crossfield, T. (1990) The CPN and depot injections. *Journal of Clinical Practice, Education and Management*, **4**(13), 24–5.

Dean, E. (1988) *Evaluation of Community Psychiatric Nursing Service in Tunbridge Wells Health Authority*, Research Monograph, Bexley Health Authority, Bexley.

Dick, D. (1986) Mental health nursing: why change? *Nursing Times*, **January**, 55–6.

Dickers, A. and Callaghan, P. (1992) CPNs and adults sexually absued in childhood. *Nursing times*, **88**(4), 45.

Dickinson, P. (1984) Can CPNs offer a more effective service to general practitioners in central Southampton. *Community Psychiatric Nursing Journal*, **4**(5), 6–10.

Everett, A. (1990) The new GP contract and community psychiatric nurses. *Community Psychiatric Nursing Journal*, **10**(6), 21–2.

Fadbadegun, R. (1985) Management of neurosis: why do the neurotics features so much in the community psychiatric nurse's work? *Community Psychiatric Nursing Journal*, **5**(1), 24–5.

Farewell, T. (1976) Crisis intervention. *Nursing Mirror*, **143**(10), 60–1.

Faugier, J. (1987) Skills and models: alone in the community. *Mental Health Nursing*, **2**, 5–6.

Faugier, J. (1992) The challenge of change: community psychiatric nursing. *Nursing Times*, **26 August**, 50–2.

Faugier, J. (1993) Human immunodeficiency virus HIV disease and drug misuse: research issues for CPNs, in *Community Psychiatric Nursing: A Research Perspective*, vol 2, (eds C. Brooker and E. White), Chapman & Hall, London.

Ferguson, K. (1993) A study to investigate the views of patients and their carers on the work undertaken by nurses to prepare the patient for discharge from hospital, in *Community Psychiatric Nursing: A Research Perspective*, vol. 2 (eds C. Brooker and E. White), Chapman & Hall, London.

Field, R. (1993) Patients' and CPNs' views of a CPN service, in *Community Psychiatric Nursing: A Research Perspective*, vol. 2, (eds C. Brooker and E. White), Chapman & Hall, London.

Fretwell, A. (1992) Collaboration in mental health: the role of the CPN in primary health care team. *Practice Nursing*, **May**, 18–19.

Furlong, R. (1973) Community psychiatry. *Health and Social Services Journal*, **83**, 1137–8.

Ganzevoort, J. (1975) New tasks for psychiatric nurses. *International Nursing Review*, **22**, 109–12.

George, P. and Dudley, M. (1986) Problem solving skills for chronic psychiatric patients. *Community Psychiatric Nursing Journal*, **6**(4), 8–12.

Gillam, T. (1989) Psychiatric nursing in the community. *Nursing Standard*, **4**, 25.

Gournay, K. (1991) The base for exposure treatment in agrophobia: some indicators for nurse therapists and community psychiatric nurses. *Journal of Advanced Nursing*, **16**(1), 82–91.

Gournay, K. and Brooking, J. (1992) *An Evaluation of the Effectiveness of Community Psychiatric Nurses in Treating Patients with Minor Mental Disorders in Primary Care*, Final Report to the Department of Health, HMSO, London.

Gournay, K. and Brooking, J. (1993) Failure and dissatisfaction, in *Community Psychiatric Nursing: A Research Perspective*, vol. 2, (eds C. Brooker and E. White), Chapman & Hall, London.

Greene, J. (1968) The improved outlook in psychiatry and psychiatric nursing. *Nursing Mirror*, **126**, 40.

Greene, J. (1968) The psychiatric nurse in the community nursing service. *International Journal of Nursing Studies*, **5**, 175–84.

Greene, J. (1978) Discharge and be damned: the nurse's response. *Royal Society of Health Journal*, **98**(3), 104–7.

Greenfield, C. (1980) Community psychiatric nursing: child psychiatric day centres. *Nursing Times*, **76**(24), 1064–5.

Hally, H. (1992) Community psychiatric nursing. *Openmind*, **August/September**, 20–1.

Harrigan, P., Sorensen, J. and Ryder, S. (1993) Clinical audit and CPN services, in *Community Psychiatric Nursing: a Research Perspective*, vol. 2, (eds C. Brooker and E. White), Chapman & Hall, London.

Hassell, C. and Stilwell, J. (1978) *The Work of the Community Psychiatric Nursing Service: Worcester Development Project Research and Development Report No. 3*, Birmingham University Health Services Research Unit, Birmingham.

Hess, G. (1971) Between two worlds (community mental health nursing in the USA). *International Journal of Nursing Studies*, **8**, 37–46.

Higginson, A. (1983) *An Exploratory Study to Evaluate Community Psychiatric Nurses' Attitudes Toward Particular Diagnostic and Age Categories*, Research Monograph, Manchester Polytechnic, Manchester.

Horrock, P. (1985) *Memorandum to Social Services Committee on Community Care, with Special Reference to Adult Mentally Ill and Mentally Handicapped People (on Behalf of the NHS Health Advisory Service)*, HMSO, London.

Howson, D., Malkin, J. and Munslow, G. (1989) Working with the elderly functionally ill with a mobile day hospital. *Community Psychiatric Nursing Journal*, **9**(5), 24–5.

Hudson, B. (1975) A behaviour modification project with chronic schizophrenics in the community. *Behaviour Research and Therapy*, **13**(4), 339–41.

Hughes, C. (1991) Community psychiatric nursing and the depressed patient: a case for using cognitive therapy. *Journal of Advanced Nursing*, **16**(5), 565–72.

Hughes, C. (1992) Community psychiatric nursing and depression in elderly people. *Journal of Advanced Nursing*, **17**(1), 34–42.

Hughes, C. (1992) Prevalence and prognosis of depression in elderly people: implications for CPN practice. *Community Psychiatric Nursing Journal*, **12**(4), 7–11.

Hughes, C. (1993) A review of a psychological intervention for depression in elderly people, in *Community Psychiatric Nursing: a Research Perspective*, vol. 2, (eds C. Brooker and E. White), Chapman & Hall, London.

Hugo, M., Goldney, R., Skinner, E. *et al.* (1984) Using screening instruments in community psychiatric nursing for the elderly. *Australian Journal of Advanced Nursing*, **2**(2), 13–17.

Hunter, P. (1962) Aftercare for the mentally ill as one British hospital provides it. *Nursing Outlook*, **10**(9), 604–6.

Hunter, P. (1978) *Schizophrenia and Community Psychiatric Nursing*, National Schizophrenia Fellowship, Surbiton, Surrey.

Imlah, N. and Murphy, K. (1976) A planned system of community care for schizophrenia in Great Britain. *Australian and New Zealand Journal of Psychiatry*, **10**(2), 141–5.

Irish Journal of Psychiatric Nursing (1980) Whither community psychiatric nursing? *Irish Journal of Psychiatric Nursing*, **January**, 32–3.

Jarvis, J. (1990) *Report of Community Psychiatric Nursing Survey*, Wessex Regional Health Authority, Winchester.

Jebali, C. (1991) Working together to support women with depression: collaboration between health visitors and community psychiatric nurses. *Health Visitor*, **64**(12), 410–11.

Jones, A. (1989) Liaison consultation psychiatry: the CPN as clinical nurse specialist. *Community Psychiatric Nursing Journal*, **9**(2), 7–14.

Knowles, K. (1990) *Evaluation of the Community Psychiatric Nursing Service in Burnley, Pendle and Rossendale 1989–1990*, Research Monograph, Department of Nursing, University of Manchester, Manchester.

Koldjeski, D. (1984) *Community Mental Health Nursing: New Directions in Theory and Practice*, John Wiley, New York.

Laird, D. (1978) *Report of a Survey to Determine the Need for Psychiatric Nursing Services Within Primary Health Care Teams*, Nottingham Area Health Authority, Nottingham.

Lancaster, J. (1979) Community treatment for mental health's forgotten population in USA. *Journal of Psychiatric Nursing*, **17**(7), 20–7.

Leopoldt, H. (1973) Psychiatric community nursing. *Health and Social Services Journal*, **83**, 489–90.

Leopoldt, H. (1975) Community psychiatric nursing. *Nursing Times* (Occasional Paper) **74**, 13–14.

Leopoldt, H. (ed.) (1978) *Contemporary Themes in Psychiatric Nursing*, Squibb & Son, Twickenham.

Leopoldt, H., Corea, S. and Robinson, R. (1975) Hospital-based community psychiatric nursing in psychogeriatric care. *Nursing Mirror*, **141**(25), 54–6.

Leopoldt, H. and Hurn, R. (1973) Psychiatric nurse in the community. *Practice Team*, **21**, 2–4.

Llewellyn, E. (1974) Community psychiatric nursing. *Midwives and Health Visitors Journal*, **10**, 7–9.

MacDonald, L. (1990) Community mental health services from the users perspective: an evaluation of the Doddington Edward Wilson mental health services. *International Journal of Social Psychiatry*, **36**(3), 183–93.

McDonnell, D. (1977) An evaluation of day centre care. *International Journal of Social Psychiatry*, **23**(2), 110–19.

McFadyen, J. (1985) Primary health care attachment and primary prevention vs. hospital attachment and generic prevention. *Community Psychiatric Nursing Journal*, **5**(3), 30–7.

McKendrick, D. (1984) Weekend working: a survey of community psychiatric nursing services in the North West Region. *Community Psychiatric Nursing Journal*, **4**(6), 7–12.

MacLeod, W. (1970) Domiciliary psychiatric nursing observed. *Nursing Times*, (Occasional Paper), **66**(50), 185–90.

Major, S. (1993) Attitudes towards supervision: a comparison between CPNs and managers, in *Community Psychiatric Nursing: A Research Perspective*, vol. 2, (eds C. Brooker and E. White), Chapman & Hall, London.

Manchester, J. (1983) A framework for planning: the introduction of the nursing process into a community psychiatric nursing setting. *Nursing Mirror*, **156**(15), 34–6.

Mangen, S. and Griffith, J. (1982) Patient satisfaction with community psychiatric nursing: a prospective controlled study. *Journal of Advanced Nursing*, **7**(5), 477–82.

Mann, P. (1979) How a nurse taught doctors psychiatry. *General Practitioner*, **August**, 31.

Marks, I. (1975) A symposium on the psychiatric nurse-therapist: A new form of clinical nurse specialist. *Nursing Mirror*, **140**(19), 46.

Marks, I. (1985) *Psychiatric Nurse Therapists in Primary Care: The Expansion of Advanced Clinical Roles in Nursing*, Royal College of Nursing, London.

Matthews, L. (1990) A role for the CPN in supporting the carer of clients with dementia, in *Community Psychiatric Nursing: A Research Perspective*, (ed. C. Brooker), Chapman & Hall, London.

May, A. (1965) The psychiatric nurse in the community. *Nursing Mirror*, **120**, 409–10.

May, A. and Moore, S. (1963) The mental nurse in the community. *Lancet*, **i**, 213–14.

Mellor, P. (1987) Compulsory treatment in the community. *Nursing Standard*, **7 May**, 5.

Mercer, B. and Brough, R. (1987) Compulsory treatment in the community: a local survey of CPNs. *Community Psychiatric Nursing Journal*, **7**(4), 16–18.

Meredith-Smith, P. (1990) Harm reduction schemes for injecting drug users: ethical dilemmas for CPNs. *Community Psychiatric Nursing Journal*, **10**(5), 8–13.

Milne, D., Walker, J. and Bentnick, V. (1985) The value of feedback: an example of evaluation research in community psychiatric nursing care. *Nursing Times*, **81**, 34–6.

Minghella, E. (1989) The role of the nurse in the management of parasuicide in the community, in *Directions in Nursing Research: Ten Years of Progress at London University*, (eds J. Wilson-Barnett and S. Robinson), Scutari, Harrow.

Moore, S. (1961) A psychiatric outpatient nursing service. *Mental Health Bulletin*, **20**, 51–4.

Moore, S. (1964) Mental nursing in the community. *Nursing Times*, **10**(60), 467–70.

Morrall, P. (1992) Transferable skills and community psychiatric nursing. *Community Psychiatric Nursing Journal*, **12**(5), 14–18.

Munton, R. (1990) Client satisfaction with community psychiatric nursing, in *Community Psychiatric Nursing: A Research Perspective*, (ed. C. Brooker), Chapman & Hall, London.

Nursing Mirror (1976) Community psychiatric nursing. *Nursing Mirror* (JBCNS Supplement 2), **5 August**.

O'Hanlon, P. (1987) Team approach soothes GP fears and improves services. *Geriatric Medicine*, **17**(2), 43–6.

Oltman, P. (1971) One approach to real community involvement. *Journal of Psychiatric Nursing*, 9(5), 18–21.

Osborne, A. (1970) A theoretical basis for the education of the psychiatric mental health nurse. *Nursing Clinics of North America*, 5(4), 699–712.

Parahoo, K. and Robinson, G. (1989) CPNs in Northern Ireland 1. *Senior Nurse*, 9(10), 12–14.

Parahoo, K. and Robinson, G. (1990) CPNs in Northern Ireland 2. *Senior Nurse*, 10(1), 24–7.

Parahoo, K. and Robinson, G. (1990) CPNs in Northern Ireland 3. *Senior Nurse*, 10(2), 20–4.

Parnell, J. (1974) Psychiatric nursing in the community. *Queen's Nursing Journal*, 27(2), 36–8.

Parry, J. (1991) Community care and mentally ill offenders. *Nursing Standard*, 5(23), 29–33.

Paykel, E. and Griffith, J. (1983) *Community Psychiatric Nursing: the Springfield Controlled Trial*, Royal College of Nursing, London.

Paykel, E., Mangen, S., Griffith, J. and Burns, T. (1982) Community psychiatric nursing for neurotic patients: a controlled trial. *British Journal of Psychiatry*, **June**, 573–81.

Peat, L. (1979) Twenty five years of community psychiatric nursing. *Community Psychiatric Nurses Association Journal*, **January**.

Phillips, M. (1978) Joint planning and shared responsibility. *Social Work Services*, 15, 28–31.

Pierloot, R. and Demarsin, M. (1981) Family care versus hospital stay for chronic psychiatric patients. *International Journal of Social Psychiatry*, 27(3), 217–24.

Pollock, L. (1986) An evaluation research study of Community Psychiatric Nursing, employing the Personal Questionnaire Rapid Scaling Technique. *Community Psychiatric Nursing Journal*, 6(3), 11–21.

Pollock, L. (1987) Community psychiatric nursing explained: an analysis of the views of patients, carers and nurses. University of Edinburgh, PhD Thesis.

Pollock, L. (1988) The work of community psychiatric nursing. *Journal of Advanced Nursing*, 13(5), 537–45.

Pollock, L. (1990) The goals and objectives of community psychiatric nursing, in *Community Psychiatric Nursing: A Research Perspective*, (ed. C. Brooker), Chapman & Hall, London.

Portnoy, E., Acker, S., Keithline, C. and Lewis, J. (1988) Community mental health nursing. *Journal of Gerontology Nursing*, 14(6), 13–18.

Pullen, I. (1980) Description of an extramural service for psychiatric emergencies. *Health Bulletin*, 38(4), 163–6.

Pyke-Lees, R. (1978) Care of the schizophrenic at home. *Midwife, Health Visitor and Community Nurse*, 14(9), 300–2.

Rawlinson, J. and Brown, A. (1991) Community psychiatric nursing in Britain, in *Community Psychiatry: The Principles*, (eds D. Bennett and H. Freeman), Churchill Livingstone, Edinburgh.

Redden-Lafreniere, C. (1983) Community mental health: a nursing alternative in Canada. *Canadian Journal of Psychiatric Nursing*, 24(2), 11.

Richards, D., Butterworth, G. and Shrubbs, S. (1988) Outcome measures in community psychiatric nursing: a pilot study. *Community Psychiatric Nursing Journal*, **8**(6), 7–16.

Richards, H. and Smith, H. (1970) Nursing in response to social crisis: what is community mental health in a black community? *Nursing Clinics of North America*, **5**(4), 647–55.

Rushforth, D. (1986) An evaluation of the management of deliberate self-harm in a Health Authority, using the community psychiatric nurse as an agent. Manchester Polytechnic, MPhil Thesis.

Salkovskis, R., Atha, C. and Storer, D. (1989) Defining the problem: community psychiatric nurses role attached to an Accident and Emergency Department. *Nursing Times*, **85**(44), 50–2.

Sharpe, G. (1985) Effective and efficient. *Nursing Mirror*, **16**, 39–41.

Shaw, A. (1977) CPN attachment in a group practice. *Nursing Times*, **73**(12),9–14.

Shepherd, M. (1990) Social work and community psychiatric nursing, in *The Sociology of the Caring Professions*, (eds P. Abbott and C. Wallace), Falmer Press, London.

Shepherd, M. (1991) *Mental Health Work in the Community: Theory and Practice in Social Work and Community Psychiatric Nursing*, Falmer Press, London.

Simmons, S. (1984) Community psychiatry in Bloomsbury: caught before the crisis. *Nursing Times*, **80**(44), 49–50.

Simmons, S. (1984) Family burden: what does it mean to the carers? University of Surrey, MSc Thesis.

Simmons, S. (1987) Community psychiatric nursing, in *Community Nursing*, (ed. J. Littlewood), Churchill Livingstone, Edinburgh.

Simmons, S. (1988) Community psychiatric nurses and multidisciplinary working. *Community Psychiatric Nursing Journal*, **8**(4), 14–18.

Simmons, S. (1990) Family burden: what does psychiatric illness mean to the carers? in *Community Psychiatric Nursing: A Research Perspective*, (ed. C. Brooker), Chapman & Hall, London.

Simmons, S. and Brooker, C. (1987) Making CPNs part of the team. *Nursing Times*, **83**, 49–51.

Skidmore, D. and Friend, W. (1984) Community psychiatric nursing: muddling through. *Community Outlook*, **May**, 179–81.

Skidmore, D. and Friend, W. (1984) CPNs need enrolled nurses. *Community Outlook*, **August**, 299–301.

Skidmore, D. and Friend, W. (1984) Specialism or escapism? *Community Outlook*, **September, 310–12.**

Skidmore, D. and Friend, W. (1984) Community psychiatric nursing: over to you! *Community Outlook*, **October**, 369, 371.

Sladden, S. (1975) Hospital based community psychiatric nursing service. *Nursing Mirror*, **141**(4), 56.

Sladden, S. (1979) The work of community psychiatric nurses in a hospital based community service. University of Edinburgh, PhD Thesis.

Sladden, S. (1979) *Psychiatric Nursing in the Community*, Churchill Livingstone, Edinburgh.

Slavinsky, A. and Krausa, J. (1982) Two approaches to the management of long term psychiatric outpatients in the community. *Nursing Research*, **31**(5), 284–9.

Smith, J. (1991) The Hillsborough Disaster: the personal account of a post-disaster worker. *Community Psychiatric Nursing Journal*, **11**(2), 18–23.

Social Services Committee on Community Care (1985) *Community Care with Special Reference to Adult Mentally Ill and Mentally Handicapped People, Second report (vols. 1–3)*, HMSO, London.

Spy, T. (1980) Look to the future. *Nursing Mirror*, **151**(22), 42–3.

Storer, D., Whiteworth, R., Salkovskis, P. and Atha, C. (1987) Community psychiatric nursing intervention in an Accident and Emergency Department: a clinical pilot study. *Journal of Advanced Nursing*, **12**(2), 215–22.

Stromboni, J. (1987) Home Visiting [account of work by a French CPN]. *Community Psychiatric Nursing Journal*, **7**(1), 17–19.

Strong, F. (1975) Wessex, first of its kind: CPN and alcoholism. *Nursing Times*, **71**(22), 838–40.

Strumwasser, I. (1978) The plight of the nurse in community mental health centres. *International Journal of Nursing Studies*, **15**(2), 67–73.

Swaffield, L. (1983) Community psychiatric nursing: CPNs present and future. *Community Outlook*, **August**, 219–20.

Teague, G. and Cassidy, P. (1986) Focus on Belfast: a view of community psychiatric nursing in the city. *Community Psychiatric Nursing Journal*, **6**(4), 29–30.

Thomas, M. (1989) *A Survey of Forensic Community Psychiatric Nurses*, Research Monograph, Department of Health Studies, Sheffield City Polytechnic, Sheffield.

Thompson, R. (1984) Community psychiatric nursing in Clwyd. Department of Psychiatric Social Work, University of Manchester, MSc Thesis.

Tippings, R. and White, D. (1978) New community nursing service for the elderly mentally ill. *Nursing Times*, **74**(42), 1719–20.

Tough, H., Kingerlee, P. and Elliot, P. (1980) Surgery attached psychogeriatric nurses: an evaluation of psychiatric nurses in the primary health care team. *Journal of the Royal College of General Practitioners*, **30**, 85–9.

Trotter, B. (1992) Team spirit: using community psychiatric nursing skills in a team in Oxford. *Nursing Times*, **8 July**, 33–5.

Tumility, E. (1979) Community psychiaric nursing. *Nursing Times* (Occasional Paper), **65**(40), 157–8.

Turner, G. (1993) Client/CPN contact during the administration of depot medications: implications for practice, in *Community Psychiatric Nursing: A Research Perspective*, vol. 2, (eds C. Brooker and E. White), Chapman & Hall, London.

Turner, T. (1989) CPNs and the team. *Journal of District Nursing*, **8**(3), 20–2.

Tyrer, P. and Gelder, M. (1990) The future of community psychiatric nursing: some research findings. *Psychiatric Bulletin*, **14**(9), 550–1.

Wadsworth, R. (1984) Turning point for the homeless. *Nursing Times*, **80**(44), 48.

Walgrove, N. (1986) Mental health aftercare: where is nursing? *Nursing Clinics of North America*, **21**(3), 473–81.

Walsh, P. (1976) Mental illness, mental handicap and the nursing service establishment: an alternative approach. *Journal of Advanced Nursing*, **6**, 28.

Waterreus, A. (1993) The CPN and depression in elderly people living in the community, in *Community Psychiatric Nursing: A Research Perspective*, vol. 2, (eds C. Brooker and E. White), Chapman & Hall, London.

Weeks, K. and Greene, J. (1966) Psychiatric nurses in the community. *Nursing Times*, **62**(8), 257–8.

White, E. (1986) Factors influencing general practitioners to refer patients to community psychiatric nurses, in *Psychiatric Nursing Research*, (ed. J. Brooking), John Wiley, Chichester.

White, E. (1993) Community psychiatric nursing 1980–1990: a review of organisation, education and practice, in *Community Psychiatric Nursing: A Research Perspective*, vol. 2, (eds C. Brooker and E. White), Chapman & Hall, London.

White, E. and Barker, P. (1991) The Italian experience. *Nexus*, **1**(3), 36–40.

Wilkin, P. (1988) Someone to watch over me. *Nursing Times*, **84**, 333–4.

Willey, R. (1969) Nursing after care in psychiatry. *Nursing Times*, **65**(51), 1692.

Williams, R. (1974) Team work: the key to community psychiatric nursing. *Canadian Journal of Psychiatric Nursing*, **15**, 15–17.

Woods, R. (1990) Counselling services for adolescents within a Northern Ireland community psychiatric nursing service. *Nursing Standard*, **4**, 17–19.

Wooff, K. and Goldberg, D. (1988) Further observations on the practice of community care in Salford: differences between community psychiatric nurses and mental health social workers. *British Journal of Psychiatry*, **153**, 30–7.

Wooff, K., Goldberg, D. and Fryers, T. (1988) The practice of community psychiatric nursing and mental health social work in Salford: some implications for community care. *British Journal of Psychiatry*, **152**, 783–92.

Wooff, K., Goldberg, D. and Fryers, T. (1986) Patients in receipt of community psychiatric nursing care in Salford 1976–82. *Psychological Medicine*, **16**(2), 407–14.

World Health Organization (1956) *Expert Committee on Psychiatric Nursing: First Report*, World Health Organization, Geneva.

Wright, H. (1990) Psychodynamic experience in the community. *Nursing Standard*, **4**, 32–4.

Role

Anderson, Y. (1976) Nurses' role in community psychiatry implies different requirements for psychiatric nursing. *Sygeplejersken*, **45**, 18–20.

Anonymous (1980) Royal College completes 'Role of the CPN' Report. *Community Psychiatric Nurses Association Journal*, **1**(5), 4–5.

Bagley, C. and Evan-Wong, L. (1973) The community psychiatric nurse's role and potential interest in psychiatric nursing in teenagers making a career choice. *International Journal of Nursing Studies*, **10**(4), 271–7.

Barratt, E. (1989) Community psychiatric nurses: their self-perceived roles. *Journal of Advanced Nursing*, **14**(1), 42–8.

Brandon, S. (1990) Rethinking the role of the CPN. *Nursing Times*, **86**(51), 64–6.

Brooker, C. (1990) A new role for the community psychiatric nurse in working with families caring for a relative with schizophrenia. *International Journal of Social Psychiatry*, **36**(3), 216–24.

Brooker, C. (1990) The application of the concept of expressed emotion to the role of the community psychiatric nurses: a research study. *International Journal of Nursing Studies*, **27**(3), 277–85.

Community Psychiatric Nurses Association (1978) *Role of the CPN: Evidence to Royal College of Psychiatrists*, Community Psychiatric Nurses Association, Bristol.

224 *Community psychiatric nursing: selected bibliography*

David, A. and Underwood, P. (1976) Role, function and decision making in community mental health. *Nursing Research*, **25**(4), 256–8.

Drake, W. (1981) The role of the nurse: the community psychiatric nurse, in *Handbook of Psychiatric Rehabilitation Practice*, (eds S. Wing and B. Morris), Oxford University Press, Oxford.

Flaye, A. (1990) *A Study to Examine the Role and Function of the Community Psychiatric Nurse*, Research Monograph, Royal College of Nursing, London.

Goldberg, D. (1985) Implementation of mental health policies in the North-West of England, in *The Provision of Mental Health Services in Britain: The Way Ahead*, (eds G. Wilkinson and H. Freeman), Gaskell Press, London.

Hall, V. and Russell, O. (1982) The community mental health nurse: a new professional role. *Journal of Advanced Nursing*, **7**(1), 3–10.

Harris, M. and Solomon, J. (1977) Roles of the community mental health nurse. *Journal of Psychiatric Nursing and Mental Health Services*, **15**(2), 35–9.

Joint Committee of Mental Health Nursing Organisations (1986) *The Role of the Psychiatric Nurse*. Joint Committee of Mental Health Nursing Organisations, Manchester Polytechnic, Manchester.

Leopoldt, H. (1974) The role of the psychiatric community nurse in the therapeutic team. *Nursing Mirror*, **138**(5), 70–2.

Morgan, M. (1991) Which route to the future?: developments in the community psychiatric nurses role. *Professional Nurse*, **7**(2), 127–8.

Morrall, P. (1987) Recarceration: social factors influencing admission to psychiatric institutions and the role of the community psychiatric nurse as an agent of social control. *Community Psychiatric Nursing Journal*, **7**(6), 25–32.

Nytanga, L. and McSweeny, P. (1990) Helper qualities as inner resources: the role of the CPN. *Community Psychiatric Nursing Journal*, **10**(5), 18–25.

Pederson, P. (1988) The role of the community psychiatric nurse in forensic psychiatry. *Community Psychiatric Nursing Journal*, **8**(3), 12–17.

Power, J. (1991) Expanding the role of community mental health nurses. *Canadian Nurse*, **87**(5), 20–1.

Royal College of Nursing (1966) *Investigation into the Role of the Psychiatric Nurse in the Community*, Monograph, Royal College of Nursing, London.

Sharpe, D. (1975) Role of the community psychiatric nurse. *Nursing Mirror*, **141**(16), 60–2.

Simms, J. (1985) Concepts in community care. *Community Psychiatric Nursing Journal*, **5**(6), 18–21.

Spence, G. and Baker, P. (1981) Factors affecting the performance of a prescribed community psychiatry role for nurses. *Canada's Mental Health*, **29**(4), 36–9.

Stokes, G. (1970) Extending the role of the psychiatric mental health nurse in community mental health. *Nursing Clinics of North America*, **5**(4), 635–46.

Swailes, S. (1976) Establishing good communications: experiences of a community charge nurse in establishing contact with other health professionals. *Queen's Nursing Journal*, **18**, 307–8.

Tyrer, P. (1990) Role of the community psychiatric nurse. *Nursing Times*, **86**(32), 53.

Tyrer, P., Hawksworth, J., Hobbs, R. and Jackson, D. (1990) The role of the community psychiatric nurse. *British Journal of Hospital Medicine*, **43**(6), 439–42.

Wetherill, J., Kelly, T. and Hore, B. (1987) The role of the community psychiatric nurse in improving treatment compliance in alcoholics. *Journal of Advanced Nursing*, **12**(6), 707–11.

Wilson, D. (1985) District nurse or community psychiatric nurse?' *Journal of District Nursing*, **3**(12), 25–6.

World Health Organization (1975) *Working Group on the Role of Nursing in Psychiatric and Mental Health Care*, World Health Organization, Geneva.

Worley, N. (1991) Advisor to the team: the role of the nurse in the case management approach to caring for the mentally ill in the community in the USA. *Nursing Times*, **87**, 38–40.

Social worker

Altshul, A. (1969) The role of the psychiatric nurse in the community, in *New Developments in Psychiatry and Implications for the Social Worker*, Association of Psychiatric Social Workers, London.

Arch, P. and Rajan, P. (1979) *Community Mental Health: The Role of the Community Psychiatric Nurse and the Social Worker*. University of Sussex, MA Thesis.

Barry, N. (1987) Hospital 'angels' fear their role in community care is at risk. *Social Work Today*, **19**(1), 10–11.

Brewer, C. (1983) Social workers *v.* CPNs. *Nursing Times*, **79**(24), 76.

Brook, S. (1987) Nursing and social services: collaboration or conflict? *Social Work Today*, **18**(37), 12–13.

Cole, T. (1977) Community psychiatric nursing and social work: their contributions towards community mental health services. University of Wales, Cardiff, MSc Thesis.

Donnelly, G. (1977) Relationships: the social worker and the psychiatric community nurse. *Nursing Mirror*, **145**(12), 40.

Drozd, E. and Gabell, M. (1991) Working together: cooperation of CPNs and mental health social workers. *Senior Nurse*, **11**(2), 36–40.

Hudson, B. (1976) The community psychiatric nurse and the social worker. *Nursing Times* (Community Care Supplement), **72**(21), 18–22.

Hunter, P. (1980) Social work and community psychiatric nursing: a review. *International Journal of Nursing Studies*, **17**(2), 131–9.

Manning, M. (1988) Advantage social workers. *Social Work Today*, **20**, 16–17.

Martin, F. and Kenny, W. (1979) *Patients or Clients: A Study of Social Work and Community Nursing Services for the Mentally Ill in Scotland*, Department of Social Administration, University of Glasgow, Glasgow.

Sharpe, D. (1966) The psychiatric nurse as a social visitor. *Nursing Mirror*, **62**(48), 1578–80.

Smith, T. (1969) The role of the psychiatric nurse in the community, in *New Developments in Psychiatry and the Implications for the Social Worker*, Association of Psychiatric Social Workers, London.

Wooff, K. (1986) A comparison of the roles of community psychiatric nurses and psychiatric social workers. University of Manchester, PhD Thesis.

General practitioner

Gasson, B. (1991) CPNs and general practice. *Royal College of General Practitioners Connection*, **30 June**, 2–3.

Gillespie, J. (1981) The psychiatric nurse in general practice. *Nursing Times*, **June**, 71–2.

Godin, P. and Wilson, I. (1986) Selling skills: why do so few GPs refer patients to community psychiatric nurses? *Nursing Times* (Community Outlook), 27–9.

Gournay, K., Devilly, G. and Brooker, C. (1993) The CPN in primary care: a pilot study of the process of assessment, in *Community Psychiatric Nursing: A Research Perspective*, vol. 2, (eds C. Brooker and E. White), Chapman & Hall, London.

Illing, J., Drinkwater, C., Rogerson, T. *et. al.*, (1990) Evaluation of community psychiatric nursing in general practice, in *Community Psychiatric Nursing: A Research Perspective*, (eds C. Brooker and E. White), Chapman & Hall, London.

Leopoldt, H., Hopkins, H. and Overall, R. (1974) A critical review of an experimental psychiatric nurse attachment scheme in Oxford. *Practice Team*, **39**(2), 4–6.

Marks, B. (1976) *Psychiatric Community Nurses in General Practice*, Research Monograph, University of Manchester, Manchester.

Marks, I., Lindley, P. and Waters, H. (1980) *Nurse Therapy in General Practice: Epidemiology and Efficacy*, Research Monograph, Institute of Psychiatry, London.

Oyebode, F., Gadd, E., Berry, D. et al. (1988) Community psychiatric nurses in primary care: a consumer survey. *Bulletin of the Royal College of Psychiatrists*, **12**(11), 483–5.

Parkes, C. (1974) Interdisciplinary collaboration in the field of mental health: report of a conference. *Journal of the Royal College of General Practitioners*, **24 January**, 77–80.

Ramaro, M. (1987) Community psychiatric nurses: a new role. *General Practitioner*, **5 June**, 21.

Robertson, H. and Scott, D. (1985) Community psychiatric nursing: a survey of patients and problems. *Journal of the Royal College of General Practitioners*, **35**, 130–2.

Royal College of General Practitioners (1981) *Prevention of Psychiatric Disorders in General Practice*, Royal College of General Practitioners, London.

Tough, H., Kingerlee, P. and Elliot, P. (1980) Surgery attached psychogeriatric nurses: an evaluation of psychiatric nurses in the primary health care team. *Journal of the Royal College of General Practitioners*, **30**, 85–9.

White, E. (1983) 'If it's beyond me . . .': community psychiatric nurses in relation to general practice. Department of Social Policy, Cranfield Institute, MSc Thesis.

EDUCATION

Allison, M. (1980) CPNA course. *Community Psychiatric Nurses Association Journal*, **1**(3), 6–7.

Altschul, A. (1989) One or many: should Project 2000 include more community oriented practice? *Community Psychiatric Nursing Journal*, **9**(6), 14–18.

Altschul, A. (1990) The future in trust: a response to the UKCCS discussion paper on post-registration education and practice. *Community Psychiatric Nursing Journal*, **10**(5), 14–17.

Anonymous (1984) CPNs need post basic training says UKCC. *Nursing Times*, **80**(26), 8.

Anonymous (1988) CPN training too narrow to be effective. *Nursing Times*, **84**(19), 6.

Barker, P. (1989) Bridging the gap: community psychiatric nursing and education. *Nursing Standard*, **3**(20), 22–4.

Bowers, L. (1992) CPN education survey 1991–92: recruitment to post-basic CPN Certificate courses in the UK. *Community Psychiatric Nursing Journal*, **12**(2), 16–21.

Brooker, C. (1988) Effectiveness of CPN courses. *Nursing Times*, **84**, 60.

Brooker, C. (1990) A description of clients nursed by community psychiatric nurses whilst attending English National Board Clinical Course No. 811: clarification of current role? *Journal of Advanced Nursing*, **15**(2), 155–66.

Brooker, C. (1990) A six-year follow-up study of nurses attending a course in community psychiatric nursing, in *Community Psychiatric Nursing: A Research Perspective*, (ed. C. Brooker), Chapman & Hall, London.

Brooker, C. (1990) The health education needs of families caring for a schizophrenic relative and the potential role for community psychiatric nurses. *Journal of Advanced Nursing*, **15**(9), 1092–8.

Brooker, C. and Butterworth, C. (1991) Training CPNs to deliver psychosocial intervention: the implications for a role change. *International Journal of Nursing Studies*, **28**(2), 189–200.

Brooker, C., Tarrier, N., Barrowclough, C. *et al.* (1993) Skills for CPNs working with seriously mentally ill people: the outcome of a trial of psychosocial intervention, in *Community Psychiatric Nursing: A Research Perspective*, vol. 2, (eds C. Brooker and E. White), Chapman & Hall, London.

Brooker, C. and Wiggins, R. (1983) Nurse therapist variability: the implications for selection and training. *Journal of Advanced Nursing*, **8**, 321–8.

Burnard, P. (1988) Planning and running an interpersonal skills workshop: a practical guide for community psychiatric nurses. *Community Psychiatric Nursing Journal*, **8**(3), 21–7.

Butterworth, C. (1981) Who attends community psychiatric nursing courses? *Community Psychiatric Nurses Association Journal*, **2**(2), 10–14.

Butterworth, C. (1987) Mandatory training for CPNs: an interim report. *Community Psychiatric Nursing Journal*, **7**(3), 22–5.

Butterworth, C. and Skidmore, D. (1982) Mandatory training for CPNs. *Community Psychiatric Nurses Association Journal*, **March**, 1–3.

Campbell, W., Dillon, A. and Dow, I. (1983) A case for new training: an increasing need for better definition of the CPNs task. *Nursing Mirror*, **156**(3), 42–6.

Clarke, G. (1980) Short course to disaster. *Community Psychiatric Nurses Association Journal*, **1**(4), 7–8.

Cole, E. (1971) Community psychiatric nursing course. *Nursing Mirror*, **132**(20), 16.

Community Psychiatric Nurses Association (1980) *Community Psychiatric Nurses' Education, Training and Their Needs: A Discussion Paper Prepared in Response* to the Joint Board of Clinical Nursing Studies Proposal to Establish a Shortened Course for CPNs, Community Psychiatric Nurses Association, Bristol.

Community Psychiatric Nurses Association (1983) Collated response to 'The Way Forward'. *Community Psychiatric Nursing Journal*, **3**, 42–3.

Community Psychiatric Nurses Association (1983) Mandatory training for community psychiatric nurses. *Community Psychiatric Nursing Journal*, **3**, 8–10.

Cooper, G. (1991) The issue of formal training for nurses working in psychodynamic psychotherapy. *Community Psychiatric Nursing Journal*, **11**(1), 18–22.

Damant, M. (1975) Community training for mental nurses. *Health and Social Services Journal*, **8 March**.

Davis, A. and Underwood, P. (1976) Educational preparation for community mental health nursing. *Journal of Psychiatric Nursing*, **March**, 10–15.

Dexter, G. and Morrall, P. (1987) All dressed up and nowhere to go: implications for the future of CPN education. *Community Psychiatric Nursing Journal*, **7**(4), 1–15.

English National Board (1985) *Course 811: Nursing Care of Mentally Ill People in the Community for Nurses on Part 3 of the Professional Register (RMN), Notes on Outline Curricula*, English National Board for Nursing, Midwifery and Health Visiting, London.

English National Board (1989) *Course 812: Nursing Care of Mentally Ill People in the Community for Nurses on Part 3 of the Professional Register (RMN), Notes on Outline Curricula*, English National Board for Nursing, Midwifery and Health Visiting, London.

Erickson, G. (1987) Peer evaluation as a teaching-learning strategy in baccalaureate education for community mental health nursing. *Journal of Nurse Education*, **26**(5), 204–6.

Hallam, R. (1975) The training of nurse therapists. *Nursing Mirror*, **140**(19), 48–50.

Harries, C. (1972) *Psychiatric Community Care and the Psychiatric Nurse: a Discussion Paper to the Joint Board of Clinical Nursing Studies*, Joint Board of Clinical Nursing Studies, London.

Hunter, P. (1970) *The Role of the Psychiatric Nurse: Some Thoughts on Training, Briefing paper to Clinical Serices Committee*, National Association for Mental Health, London.

Joint Committee of Mental Health Nursing Organisations (1987) Mandatory training for community psychiatric nurses: an interim report. *Community Psychiatric Nursing Journal*, **7**(3), 22–5.

Joint Committee of Mental Health Nursing Organisations (1987) Mandatory training for community psychiatric nurses: a final report. *Community Psychiatric Nursing Journal*, **7**(6), 33–42.

Joint Board of Clinical Nursing Studies (1974) *Course 800: Outline Curriculum in Community Psychiatric Nursing for Registered Nurses*, Joint Board of Clinical Nursing Studies, London.

Joint Board of Clinical Nursing Studies (1979) *Course 810: Outline Curriculum in the Nursing Care of the Mentally Ill in the Community*, Joint Board of Clinical Nursing Studies, London.

Kratz, C. (1982) Properly prepared: mandatory training for CPNs. *Community Psychiatric Nurses Association Journal*, **March**, 1.

Lim, J. (1981) Mandatory training for CPNs. *Nursing Times*, **77**(52), 2237.

Milne, D. and Matanga, R. (1985) A short course in anxiety management for student psychiatric nurses during their community training. *Community Psychiatric Nursing Journal*, **5**(6), 7–12.

Nursing Times (1973) Training the psychiatric nurse of the future. *Nursing Times*, **69**, 346–8.

Nyatanga, L. (1989) The Q sort theory and technique (in relation to CPN course 811). *Nurse Education Today*, **9**(5), 347–50.

Pai, S. and Nagarajaiah, H. (1984) Treatment of schizophrenic patients in their homes through a visting nurse: some issues in nurse training. *International Journal of Nursing Studies*, **19**(3), 167–72.

Persaud, T. (1985) The general student in the community. *Community Psychiatric Nursing Journal*, **5**(1), 6–10.

Rawlings, J. (1970) Course in community psychiatry. *Nursing Mirror*, **130**(26), 20.

Rushforth, D. (1985) Mandatory training for community psychiatric nurses; Report of a conference. *Community Psychiatric Nursing Journal*, **5**(4), 3–5.

Rushforth, D. (1988) Market forces and community psychiatric nursing courses. *Community Psychiatric Nursing Journal*, **8**(6), 22–6.

Rushforth, D. (1990) Recruitment to post-basic CPN Certificate courses in the United Kingdom for 1989/90. *Community Psychiatric Nursing Journal*, **10**(2), 17–20.

Simmons, S. (1989) An exercise in (CPN) curriculum development: the process of putting theory into practice. *Nurse Education Today*, **9**(5), 327–34.

Skidmore, D. (1985) More than chalk and talk. *Community Outlook*, **September**, 11–13.

Skidmore, D. and Friend, W. (1984) Community psychiatric nursing: student rethink needed. *Community Outlook*, **July**, 258–60.

Speight, I. (1976) JBCNS course 800 in community psychiatric nursing. *Nursing Mirror*, **5 August**, 2–3.

Speight, I. (1978) Nurse education: signposts for the future, in *Contemporary Themes in Psychiatric Nursing*, (ed. H. Leopoldt), Squibb & Son, Twickenham.

Standing Advisory Group for Community Psychiatric Nursing Education (1991) *Response to the Department of Health Document 'Services for People with Mental Illnesses': A Report of a Series of Meetings with Heads of Psychiatric Nursing Services within Regional Health Authorities in England*, School of Advanced Nursing, North East Surrey College of Technology, Surrey.

Thain, A. (1976) A course member's view. *Nursing Mirror* (JBCNS supplement) **143**, 6.

Wallace, M. (1992) Forthcoming changes in post-registration and practice. *Community Psychiatric Nursing Journal*, **12**(3), 26–8.

Welsh National Board for Nursing, Midwifery and Health Visiting (1988) *Foundation Course of Preparation for Community Mental Health Nursing*, Welsh National Board for Nursing, Midwifery and Health Visiting, Cardiff.

White, E. (1981) Mandatory training for CPNs (letter). *Nursing Times*, **23 December**, 2237.

White, E. (1989) Italian community mental health services and nurse education. *Community Psychiatry: Its Practice and Management*, **1**(1), 6–8.

White, E. (1990) Historical development of the educational preparation of community psychiatric nurses, in *Community Psychiatric Nursing: a Research Perspective*, (ed. C. Brooker), Chapman & Hall, London.

230 *Community psychiatric nursing: selected bibliography*

White, E. and Brooker, C. (1990) The Standing Advisory Group for Community Psychiatric Nursing Education: grasping the nettle? *Nurse Education Today*, **February**, 63–5.

Wolsey, P. (1984) Is there a case for training CPNs in social interventions in the families of schizophrenic patients? University of Birmingham, MsocSci Thesis.

Wolsey, P. and Betts, A. (1988) What can we do with the learners? *Community Psychiatric Nursing Journal*, **8**(1), 5–12.

ORGANIZATION

Beard, P. (1981) The management and development of community nursing services for the mentally ill and the mentally handicapped. *Community Psychiatric Nurses Association Journal*, **November**, 5–9.

Black, E. and Bajoonauth, R. (1985) Shaping the future pattern of community mental health nursing services. *Nursing Practice*, **1**(1), 43–50.

Black, E., Moore, R. and Whitehead, T. (1986) A psychiatric service almost without a psychiatric hospital. *Bulletin of the Royal College of Psychiatrists*, **10**(2), 29–31.

Brooker, C. (1987) An investigation into the factors influencing variation in the growth of community psychiatric nursing services. *Journal of Advanced Nursing*, **12**(3), 367–75.

Brooker, C. and Simmons, S. (1985) A study to compare two models of community psychiatric nursing care delivery. *Journal of Advanced Nursing*, **10**(3), 217–33.

Carlisle, D. (1992) Planning the future: community psychiatric nurses in Bath prepare for change to be implemented in April 1993. *Nursing Times*, **88**(31), 38–9.

Chamberlain, J. (1983) The role of the Federal Government in the development of psychiatric nursing in the USA. *Journal of Psychosocial Nursing and Mental Health Services*, **19**(9), 15–20.

Community Psychiatric Nurses Association (1981) *Community Psychiatric Nursing Services Directory*, Community Psychiatric Nurses Assocation, Ashton in Makerfield.

Community Psychiatric Nurses Association (1985) *The CPNA/Lundbeck Directory of Community Psychiatric Nursing Services 1985–86*, CPNA Publications, Bristol.

Corea, S. (1984) Developing psychiatric services for the elderly. *Community Psychiatric Nursing Journal*, **4**(1), 5–10.

Corser, G. and Ryce, S. (1977) Community mental health care: a model based on the primary care system. *British Medical Journal*, **2**, 936–8.

Dick, D. and Mandy, C. (1989) Improving the organisation of services for the elderly mentally ill. *Geriatric Medicine*, **19**(1), 14–17.

Dixon, K. (1985) The future development of community psychiatric nursing requires an identifiable philosophy. *Community Psychiatric Nursing Journal*, **5**(2), 30–3.

Dunnell, K. and Dobbs, J. (1982) *Nurses Working in the Community*, HMSO, London.

Good Practices in Mental Health (1989) *Mental Health in Primary Care: Examples of Professional Attachments*, Good Practices in Mental Health, London.

Harker, P., Leopoldt, H. and Robinson, J. (1976) Attaching community psychiatric nurses in general practice. *Journal of the Royal College of General Practitioners*, **26**(170), 666–71.

Hunter, D. (1975) Organisational problems in community psychiatric programmes. *Journal of Psychiatric Nursing*, **16**(3), 8–11.

Lee, H. (1990) Out-of-hours work by CPNs, in *Community Psychiatric Nursing: A Research Perspective*, (ed. C. Brooker), Chapman & Hall, London.

MacKinnon, R. (1981) *A Study of Community Psychiatric Nursing Manpower Planning*, Research Monograph, Department of Molecular and Life Sciences, Dundee College of Technology, Dundee.

Martin, F. (1984) Community psychiatric nursing: filling the gap? in *Between the Acts: Community Mental Health Services 1959–1983* (ed. F. Martin), Nuffield Provincial Hospitals Trust, London.

McIntegart, J. (1982) The shape of things to come. *Nursing Times*, **78**(32), 1344–5.

Moffett, M. (1988) Evolution of psychiatric community care. *Journal of Psychosocial Nursing and Mental Health Services*, **26**(7), 17–21.

Morgan, M. (1992) The community psychiatric nursing service of the 1990s. *Community Psychiatric Nursing Journal*, **12**(1), 25–7.

Northern Ireland Association for Mental Health (1984) *Mental Health Services in Northern Ireland: A Statistical Review*, Northern Ireland Association for Mental Health, Belfast.

Pope, B. (1985) Psychiatry in transition: implications for psychiatric nursing. *Community Psychiatric Nursing Journal*, **5**(4), 7–13.

Roy, S. (1990) *Nursing in the Community: Report of the Working Group*, North West Thames Regional Health Authority, London.

Schafer, T. (1992) CPN stress and organisational change: a study. *Community Psychiatric Nursing Journal*, **12**(1), 16–24.

Scott, R. (1980) A family oriented psychiatric service to the London Borough of Barnet. *Health Trends*, **3**(12), 65–8.

Sencicle, L. (1981) Which way the CPN? *Community Psychiatric Nurses Association Journal*, **2**(1), 10–14.

Sencicle, L. (1980) Out of the wards: review of research on community psychiatric nursing and possible future directions for the service. *Nursing Mirror*, **151**(8), 40–2.

Skidmore, D. (1986) The effectiveness of community psychiatric nursing teams and base locations, in *Psychiatric Nursing Research*, (ed. J. Brooking), John Wiley, Chichester.

Stephens, M. (1984) Some methodological issues in the study of community psychiatric services. *Community Psychiatric Nursing Journal*, **4**(4), 23–6.

Whitby, P., Rule, J. and Joomratty, J. (1990) Support and stay: an innovative community service for the elderly confused. *Psychiatric Bulletin*, , **14**(12), 708–10.

White, E. (1987) Psychiatrist influence on commmunity psychiatric services planning and development and its implications for community psychiatric nurses. Department of Sociology, University of Surrey, MSc Thesis.

White, E. (1989) Chinese whispers: the folklore of community psychiatric nursing manpower planning targets. *Journal of Advanced Nursing*, **14**, 373–5.

White, E. (1990) Psychiatrists influence on the development of community psychiatric nursing services, in *Community Psychiatric Nursing: A Research Perspective*, (ed. C. Brooker), Chapman & Hall, London.

White, E. (1990) *The National Directory of Community Psychiatric Nursing Services*, CPNA Publications, Bradford.

White, E. (1990) The work of the Community Psychiatric Nurses Association: a survey of the membership. *Community Psychiatric Nursing Journal*, **10**(2), 30–5.

Wooff, K., Freeman, H. and Fryers, T. (1983) Psychiatric service use in Salford: a comparison of point prevalence ratios, 1968 and 1978. *British Journal of Psychiatry*, **142**, 588–97.

OTHER

Adams, T. (1992) The ideology that underpins community care: the implications for CPNs. *Senior Nurse*, **12**(4), 34–7.

Allum, L. (1990) Medicines administered by community psychiatric nurses: their funding sources and their effect. *Community Psychiatric Nursing Journal*, **10**(6), 16–20.

Anonymous (1978) CPNA highlights policy gap. *Community Outlook*, **August**, 213.

Anonymous (1991) 1991 National Training Conference 'Preparing for Europe' Report of Opening Address given by Yvonne Moores, Chief Nurse for Scotland. *Community Psychiatric Nursing Journal*, **11**(3), 35–6.

Atha, C., Salkovskis, P. and Storer, D. (1989) More questions than answers. *Nursing Times*, **85**(15), 28–31.

Atha, C., Salkovskis, P. and Storer, D. (1989) Problem solving treatment. *Nursing Times*, **85**, 45–7.

Australian Nurses Journal (1972) Trends in European psychiatric nursing care. *Australian Nursing Journal*, **12**, 18–19.

Baker, F. and Howard, L. (1975) Mental health ideologies of psychiatric nurses. *Community Mental Health Journal*, **11**(2), 195–202.

Barker, P. (1988) Reasoning about madness, the long search for the vanishing horizon. *Community Psychiatric Nursing Journal*, **8**(4), 7–13.

Barker, P. (1988) Reasoning about madness: the long search for the vanishing horizon. *Community Psychiatric Nursing Journal*, **8**(5), 14–19.

Barratt, E. (1989) Addicted clients: socially or mentally ill? CPNs perceptions of illness models of addiction. University of Surrey, MSc Thesis.

Boodhna, G. (1988) A survey of Scottish community psychiatric nursing services, 1988. *Community Psychiatric Nursing Journal*, **10**(6), 9–15.

Bowers, L. (1991) Much ado about nothing: publication trends in the Community Psychiatric Nursing Journal. *Community Psychiatric Nursing Journal*, **11**(5), 8–14.

Bowers, L. (1992) A preliminary description of the United Kingdom community psychiatric nursing literature, 1960–1990. *Journal of Advanced Nursing*, **17**(6), 739–46.

Bowers, L. (1992) Ethnomethodology: a study of the community psychiatric nurse in the patients home. *International Journal of Nursing Studies*, **29**(1), 69–79.

Brook, A. (1978) An aspect of community mental health consultative work with general practice teams. *Health Trends*, **10**, 37–9.

Brooker, C. (1984) Some problems associated with the measurement of community psychiatric nurse intervention. *Journal of Advanced Nursing*, **9**(2), 165–74.

Brooker, C. (1987) Mental health nursing: CPNs are disappointed with Cumberledge Report. *Nursing Times*, **83**(18), 64.

Brooker, C. and Brown, M. (1986) National follow-up of nurse therapists, in *Psychiatric Nursing Research*, (ed J. Brooking), John Wiley, Chichester.

Buchan, T. and Smith, R. (1989) Nursing process in community psychiatric nursing. *Australian Journal of Advanced Nursing*, **6**(3), 5–11.

Carr, P. (1984) Legal and ethical perspectives in the nursing care of the mentally ill. *Community Psychiatric Nursing Journal*, **4**(5), 14–18.

Carr, P. and Baxter, Y. (1985) Community Psychiatric Nurses Association response to the Social Services Committee report. *Community Psychiatric Nursing Journal*, **5**(3), 46–8.

Carr, P., Butterworth, C. and Hodges, B. (1980) *Community Psychiatric Nursing: Caring for the Mentally Ill and Handicapped in the Community*, Churchill Livingstone, Edinburgh.

Channock, A. (1979) *Should the Community Psychiatric Nurse Become a Member of the Primary Health Care Team?* Research Monograph, Royal College of Nursing, London.

Church, O. (1987) From custody to community in psychiatric nursing. *Nursing Research*, **36**(1), 48–55.

Clarke, G. (1982) Professional insecurity: lack of official recognition of community psychiatric nurses. *Nursing Mirror*, **155**(15), 31–3.

Cohen, D. (1978) Psychiatry at home. *New Statesman*, **2 March**.

Community Psychiatric Nurses Association (1978) *Carriage and Care of Drugs in the Community by CPNs*, Community Psychiatric Nurses Association, Bristol.

Community Psychiatric Nurses Association (1985) CPNA policy statement on the closure of large mental hospitals in England and Wales. *Community Psychiatric Nursing Journal*, **5**(5), 44–5.

Community Psychiatric Nurses Association (1985) Evidence to the Community Nursing Review. *Community Psychiatric Nursing Journal*, **5**(5), 36–43.

Community Psychiatric Nurses Assocation (1986) *Guidelines for Supervision*, CPNA Publications, London.

Community Psychiatric Nurses Association (1987) CPNA position paper: Community Treatment Orders. *Community Psychiatric Nursing Journal*, **7**(5), 44–5.

Community Psychiatric Nurses Association (1987) CPNA response to Community Nursing Review. *Community Psychiatric Nursing Journal*, **7**(1), 40–5.

Community Psychiatric Nurses Association (1989) *Patients Case: Views from Experience Living Inside and Out of a Psychiatric Hospital*, CPNA Publications, Bradford.

Community Psychiatric Nurses Association (1989) *Future Arrangements in Community Care: CPNA Response to Recent Policy Statements*, CPNA Publications, Bradford.

Cooper, G. (1989) The usefulness of the concept of preventive mental health to the community psychiatric nurse. *Community Psychiatric Nursing Journal*, **9**(1), 7–11.

Corrigan, J. (1989) The concept of the sick role, with particular reference to the community psychiatric nursing team. *Community Psychiatry*, **1**(4), 45–6.

Dawe, A-M. (1979) The saving figures: how Shenley's community psychiatric nursing service saves money. *Community View*, **December**, 2.

Dawe, A-M. (1980) A case for community psychiatric nurses. *Journal of Advanced Nursing*, **5**(5), 485–90.

Dawe, A-M. (1980) To be or not to be: an assessment to evaluate if community psychiatric nurses give value for money. *Community Psychiatric Nurses Association Journal*, **February**, 10–12.

Dibner, L. and Murphy, J. (1991) Nurse entrepreneurs: community based programme for chronically mentally ill people, involving self-employed nurses. *Journal of Psychosocial Nursing and Mental Health Services*, **29**(3), 30–4.

Driver, E. (1976) *Assess Demand for Community Psychiatric Nursing Services in Chester District and Pinpoint Possible Growth Areas*, Research Monograph, Manchester Polytechnic, Manchester.

Etherington, S. (1984) Community mental health workers: Canadian developments could be used in a model for Britain. *Openmind*, **11**, 12.

Fear, C. and Wilkinson, G. (1992) Prescribing community psychiatric nurses. *Psychiatric Bulletin*, **16**(2), 76–7.

Feinmann, J. (1985) An CPN experiment paying dividends. *Health and Social Services Journal*, **95** (4968), 1228–9.

Ferguson, G. (1992) Race and mental health. *Community Psychiatric Nursing Journal*, **12**(6), 11–17.

Gasson, B. (1991) Community psychiatric nursing: looking into the past. *Community Psychiatric Nursing Journal*, **11**(4), 17–21.

Giles, P. (1990) Standards for community psychiatric nursing services. *Community Psychiatric Nursing Journal*, **10**(4), 8–12.

Gillam, T. (1991) 'Community' and 'Neighbourhood': how concepts shape the provision of care. *Community Psychiatric Nursing Journal*, **11**(4), 12–16.

Greene, J. (1989) The beginnings of community psychiatric nursing. *History of Nursing Group at the Royal College of Nursing Bulletin*, **2**(9), 14–20.

Griffith, J. and Mangen, S. (1980) Community psychiatric nursing: a literature review. *International Journal of Nursing Studies*, **17**, 197–210.

Handyside, L. and Heyman, B. (1990) Community mental health care: clients perceptions of services and an evaluation of a voluntary agency support scheme. *International Journal of Social Psychiatry*, **36**(4), 280–90.

Hardy-Price, D. (1990) Technology and the CPN. *Nursing* **4**(10), 16–18.

Harris, M. (1992) A comparative review of the Framework for Dynamic Standard Setting and Audit of Nursing Services FANS in the context of community psychiatric nursing. *Community Psychiatric Nursing Journal*, **12**(5), 7–13.

Hawks, K. (1975) Community care: an analysis of assumptions. *British Journal of Psychiatry*, **127**, 276–85.

Henden, J. (1985) The case for small caseloads. *Community Psychiatric Nursing Journal*, **5**(1), 18–19.

Hill, J. (1989) Supervision in the caring professions: a literature review. *Community Psychiatric Nursing Journal*, **9**(5), 9–15.

Hilton, B (1990) A health education package for schizophrenic sufferers and their families and friends. *Community Psychiatric Nursing Journal*, **10**(4), 22–9.

Howard, L. and Baker, F. (1971) Ideology and role function of the nurse in community mental health. *Nursing Research*, **20**, 450–4.

Hunter, P. (1959) *The Changing Function of Professional Staff in the Mental Hospital, Ventures in Professional Cooperation*, Association of Psychiatric Social Workers, London.

Hunter, P. (1974) Community psychiatric nursing in Britain: an historical review. *International Journal of Nursing Studies*, **11**, 223–33.

Hunt, M. and Mangan, J. (1990) Information for practice through computerised records, in *Community Psychiatric Nursing: A Research Perspective*, (ed. C. Brooker), Chapman & Hall, London.

International Council of Nurses (1990) *The Current Status of Psychiatric/Mental Health Nursing and Future Changes*, International Council of Nurses, Geneva.

Khandwalla, M. (1985) A specialist community psychiatric service for ethnic minorities. *Community Psychiatric Nursing Journal*, 5(1), 20–2.

Mangen, S., Paykel, E., Griffith, J. *et al.* (1983) Cost effectiveness of community psychiatric nurse or outpatient psychiatrist care of neurotic patients. *Psychological Medicine*, 13(2), 407–16.

Marks, B. (1977) Patients referred to community psychiatric nurses. *British Medical Journal*, ii, 1154.

Marks, I., Bird, J. and Lindley, P. (1978) Behavioural nurse therapists: developments and implications. *Behavioural Psychotherapy*, 6, 25–36.

Martin, P. and James, G. (1992) Evaluating the quality of CPN care. *Community Psychiatric Nursing Journal*, 12(4), 18–21.

Miller, J. (1981) Theoretical basis for the practice of community mental health nursing. *Issues in Mental Health Nursing*, 3(4), 319–39.

Morgan, M. (1992) How should community psychiatric nurses, be graded? *Community Psychiatric Nursing Journal*, 12(2), 8–10.

Morrall, P. (1989) The professionalisation of community psychiatric nursing: a review. *Community Psychiatric Nursing Journal*, 9(4), 14–22.

Morrison, J. (1977) Differential attitudes of community agencies towards mental illness: a dilemma for the psychiatric nurse. *Journal of Psychiatric Nursing and Mental Health Services*, 15(7), 25–9.

Neely, S. (1992) 'The Worried Well': myth or reality? *Community Psychiatric Nursing Journal*, 12(4), 12–17.

Nunn, D. (1991) Opinion: community psychiatric nursing excluded from decision on compulsory admission. *Nursing Times*, 87(27), 68.

O'Reilly, R., O'Donovan, C. and Cernovsky, Z. (1990) Differences between patients', relatives' and physicians evaluations of a community psychiatric nursing program. *Journal of Community Psychology*, 18(3), 298–303.

Packham, H. (1978) *A Special Report on Caring for Psychiatric Patients by Community Psychiatric Nurses*, Confederation of Health Service Employers, London.

Parahoo, K. (1991) Job satisfaction of community psychiatric nurses in Northern Ireland. *Journal of Advanced Nursing*, 16(3), 317–24.

Parrish, D. (1985) Sociology and the community psychiatric nurse. *Community Psychiatric Nursing Journal*, 5(5), 9–12.

Parrish, D. (1987) Health education and community psychiatric nursing. *Community Psychiatric Nursing Journal*, 7(5), 11–15.

Pollock, L. (1988) The future work of community psychiatric nursing. *Community Psychiatric Nursing Journal*, 8(5), 5–13.

Pollock, L. (1983) Community psychiatric nursing: a review and au revoir! *Community Psychiatric Nurses Association Journal*, 3(3), 30–6.

Rankin, H. and Slade, C. (1983) Supervision: an essential requirement for the community psychiatric nurse. *Community Psychiatric Nurses Association Journal*, 3(4), 10–14.

Rogers, B. (1986) Cumberledge: a review of the Review. *Community Psychiatric Nursing Journal*, **6**(4), 22–4.

Royal College of Psychiatrists (1980) Community psychiatric nursing: a discussion document. *Bulletin of the Royal College of Psychiatrists*, **4**(8), 117–21.

Royal College of Nursing and British Medical Association (1978) *The Duties and Position of the Nurse*, Royal College of Nursing, London.

Sencicle, L. (1987) Assessing the objectives for an economic evaluation of community psychiatric nursing care. *Community Psychiatric Nursing Journal*, **7**(3), 18–21.

Sharpe, D. (1980) Figures tell their own (CPN) story. *Nursing Mirror*, **150**(2), 34–6.

Sharpe, D. (1982) GPs views of community psychiatric nurses. *Nursing Times*, **78**(40), 1664–6.

Sheehy, B. (1990) Information for quality: designing a leaflet for users of a CPN service. *Community Psychiatric Nursing Journal*, **10**(1), 24–7.

Simmons, S. and Brooker, C. (1986) *Community Psychiatric Nursing: a Social Perspective*, Heinemann, London.

Simmons, S. and Hally, H. (1992) Nurse prescribing: what are the implications for community psychiatric nursing? *Community Psychiatric Nursing Journal*, **12**(4), 33–7.

Simms, J. and Carpenter, D. (1990) Mastering the art of community skills. *Nursing Times*, **86**, 40–1.

Simpson, K. (1986) Cumberledge and the CPN. *Community Psychiatric Nursing Journal*, **6**(5), 6–10.

Simpson, K. (1988) Medical power; the CPNs millstone? *Community psychiatric nursing Journal*, **8**(3), 5–11.

Simpson, K. (1989) Community psychiatric nursing: a research based profession? *Journal of Advanced Nursing*, **14**(4), 274–80.

Sladden, S. (1991) The Scottish Nursing Standards Project. *Community Psychiatric Nursing Journal*, **11**(1), 23.

Tait, J. (1992) CPNA: Stanley Moore Memorial Lecture. *Community Psychiatric Nursing Journal*, **12**(6), 7–10.

Taylor, T. (1985) Community psychiatric nursing needs counselling skills. Report of a conference. *Community Psychiatric Nursing Journal*, **5**(4), 11–14.

Thomas, B. and Brooking, J. (1991) Reactions to a new service: to assess patient satisfaction with CPN service at the Maudsley Hospital. *Journal of Clinical Practice, Education and Management*, **4**(29), 9–11.

Thompson, R. (1984) Community psychiatric nursing in Clwyd. Department of Psychiatric Social Work, University of Manchester, MSc Thesis.

Timms, C. (1985) The early days of the Community Psychiatric Nurses Association. *Community Psychiatric Nursing Journal*, **5**(5), 15–16.

Vinten, G. (1980) Community psychiatric nursing in financial perspective. *Community Psychiatric Nurses Association Journal*, **1**(3), 8–12.

Walton, J. (1984) Specialism within the community team. *Community Psychiatric Nursing Journal*, **4**(4), 29–30.

Warren, J. (1971) Long acting phenothiazine injections given by psychiatric nurses in the community. *Nursing Times* (Occasional Paper), **67**(36), 141–3.

Watt, G. (1984) The passing of an era: an interview with Lena Peat. *Community Psychiatric Nursing Journal*, **4**(2), 12–16.

White, E. (1991) Community psychiatric nurses and practice nurse: changing places. *Practice Nurse*, **4**(29), 17–19.

Whitfield, W. and Shelley, P. (1991) Violence and the CPN: a literature review. *Community Psychiatric Nursing Journal*, **11**(1), 12–17.

Whitfield, W. and Shelley, P. (1991) Violence and the CPN: a survey. *Community Psychiatric Nursing Journal*, **11**(2), 13–17.

Williams, M. (1990) GPs and CPNs attitudes to schizophrenia. *Nursing Times*, **86**(15), 53.

Index

Page numbers appearing in **bold** refer to figures and page numbers appearing in *italic* refer to tables.